THE

NEW GYMNASTICS

FOR

MEN, WOMEN, AND CHILDREN.

WITH A

TRANSLATION OF PROF. KLOSS'S DUMB-BELL INSTRUCTOR
AND PROF. SCHREBER'S PANGYMNASTIKON.

By DIO LEWIS, M. D.,
PROPRIETOR OF THE ESSEX STREET GYMNASIUM, BOSTON.

WITH THREE HUNDRED ILLUSTRATIONS.

"By no other way can men approach nearer to the gods, than by conferring health on men." — CICERO.

SEVENTH EDITION.

BOSTON:
TICKNOR AND FIELDS.
1864.

GV
481
.L67
1864

Entered according to Act of Congress, in the year 1862, by
DIO LEWIS,
in the Clerk's Office of the District Court of the District of Massachusetts.

MU

TO

THE GIRLS AND BOYS

OF AMERICA,

WHOSE PHYSICAL WELFARE HAS BEEN THE STUDY OF HIS LIFE,

THE AUTHOR

MOST AFFECTIONATELY DEDICATES

This Work.

PREFACE.

THIS book describes and illustrates a new system of physical training. Like air and food, its exercises are adapted to both sexes, and to persons of all ages.

The new system has been introduced into female seminaries with complete satisfaction. Its beautiful games, graceful attitudes, and striking tableaux, possess a peculiar fascination for girls. Public classes, composed of adults of both sexes, elicit general enthusiasm. Children under three years of age are warmly interested, and improved in form and strength.

The exercises are arranged to music, and when performed by a class, are found to possess a charm superior to that of dancing and other social amusements, while the interest increases with the skill of the performers.

This system of exercises will correct drooping or distorted shoulders, malposition of the head, and many other common defects.

Its author has been engaged many years in

teaching gymnastics. He began with a few simple exercises, and, making additions from time to time, has at length developed a very comprehensive system. Not one exercise is presented which has not been proved by long and varied use, while hundreds have been devised and rejected. Although the author has enjoyed during more than twenty years the discipline of the medical profession, its suggestions have not been adopted unless fully justified by experience in the gymnasium.

Efforts are being made to disseminate a practical knowledge of the new system. A college has been incorporated — the BOSTON NORMAL INSTITUTE FOR PHYSICAL EDUCATION, from which persons of either sex, after a full training, are graduated, with the honors of a legal diploma.

It is the ardent hope of the author that his humble labors may contribute something to the beauty and vigor of his countrymen.

CONTENTS.

THE PANGYMNASTIKON.

PHYSICAL EDUCATION.

I have nothing to say of the importance of Physical Education.

He who has not seen in the imperfect growth, pale faces, distorted forms and painful nervousness of the American People, enough to justify any and all efforts to elevate our physical tone, would not be awakened by words, written or spoken. Presuming that all who read this work are fully cognizant of the imperative need which calls it forth, I shall enter at once upon my task.

My object is to present a new system of Gymnastics. Novel in philosophy, and practical details, its distinguishing peculiarity is a complete adaptation, alike, to the strongest man, the feeblest woman, and the frailest child. The athlete finds abundant opportunities for the greatest exertions, while the delicate child is never injured.

Dispensing with the cumbrous apparatus of the ordinary gymnasium, its implements are all calculated not only to impart strength of muscle, but to give flexibleness, agility and grace of movement.

None of the apparatus, (with one or two slight exceptions,) is fixed. Each and every piece is held in the hand, so that any hall or other room may be used for the exercises.

Public Interest in Physical Education.

The true educator sees in the present public interest in physical education, a hope and a promise.

And now he is only solicitous that the great movement so auspiciously inaugurated, may not degenerate into some unprofitable speciality.

One man strikes a blow equal to five hundred pounds; another lifts eleven hundred pounds; another bends his back so that his head rests against his heels; another walks a rope over the great cataract; another runs eleven miles in an hour; another turns sixty somersets without resting.

We are greatly delighted with all these—pay our money to see them perform; but as neither one of these could do what either of the others does, so we all know that such feats, even if they were at all desirable, are not possible with one in a thousand. The question is not what shall be done for these few extraordinary persons. Each has instinctively sought and found his natural speciality.

But the question is, what shall be done for the millions of women, children and men, who are dying for physical training? My attempt to answer this momentous question will be found in this work.

DO CHILDREN REQUIRE SPECIAL GYMNASTIC TRAINING?

An eminent writer has recently declared his conviction, that boys need no studied muscle culture. "Give them," he says, "the unrestrained use of the grove, the field, the yard, the street, with the various sorts of apparatus for boys' games and sports, and they can well dispense with the scientific gymnasium."

This is a misapprehension, as is easy to convince all, who are disposed to think!

With all our lectures, conversations, newspapers,

and other similar means of mental culture, we are not willing to trust the intellect without scientific training. The poorest man in the State demands for his children the culture of the organized school; and he is right. An education left to chance and the street, would be but a disjointed product. To insure strength, patience and consistency, there must be methodical cultivation and symmetrical growth. But there is no need of argument on this point. In regard to mental training, there is, fortunately, among Americans, no difference of opinion. Discriminating, systematic, scientific culture, is our demand.

No man doubts that chess and the newspaper furnish exercise and growth; but we hold, and very justly too, that exercise and growth without qualification, are not our purpose. We require that the growth shall be of a peculiar kind—what we call scientific and symmetrical. This is vital. The education of chance would prove unbalanced, morbid, profitless.

Is not this equally true of the body? Is the body one single organ, which, if exercised, is sure to grow in the right way? On the contrary, is it not an exceedingly complicated machine, the symmetrical development of which requires discriminating, studied management? With the thoughtful mind, argument and illustration are scarcely necessary; but I may perhaps be excused by the intelligent reader for one simple illustration. A boy has round or stooping shoulders: hereby the organs of the chest and abdomen are all displaced. Give him the freedom of the yard and street—give him marbles, a ball, the skates! Does any body suppose he will become straight? Must he not, for this, and a hundred other defects have special, scientific training? There can be no doubt of it!

Before our system of education can claim an approach to perfection, we must have attached to each school a Professor, who thoroughly comprehends the wants of the body, and knows practically the means by which it may be made symmetrical, flexible, vigorous and enduring.

MILITARY DRILLS.

Since we have, unhappily, become a military people, the soldier's special training has been much considered as a means of general physical culture. Numberless schools, public and private, have already introduced the drill and make it a part of each day's exercises.

But this mode of exercise can never furnish the muscle culture which we Americans so much need. Nearly all our exercise is of the lower half of the body—we walk, we run up and down stairs, and thus cultivate hips and legs, which, as compared with the upper half of the body, are muscular. But our arms, shoulders and chests are ill-formed and weak. Whatever artificial muscular training is employed, should be specially adapted to the development of the upper half of the body.

Need I say that the military drill fails to bring into varied and vigorous play the chest and shoulders? Indeed in almost the entire drill, are not these parts held immovably in one constrained position? In all but the cultivation of uprightness, the military drill is singularly deficient in the requisites of a system of muscle training, adapted to a weak-chested people.

The exercises employed to invigorate the body,

should be such as are calculated to make the form erect, and the shoulders and chest, large and vigorous.

Dancing, to say nothing of its almost inevitably mischievous concomitants, brings into play chiefly that part of the body which is already in comparative vigor, and which, besides, has less to do directly, with the size, position and vigor of the vital organs.

Horse-back exercise is admirable, and has many peculiar advantages which can be claimed for no other training, but may it not be much indulged, while the chest and shoulders are left drooping and weak?

Skating is graceful and exhilarating, but to say nothing of the injury which not unfrequently attends the sudden change from the stagnant heat of our furnaced dwellings to the bleak winds of the icy lake, is it not true that the chest muscles are so little moved, that the finest skating may be done with the arms folded?

I suggest these thoughts for the intelligent reader, and then take the liberty to request his careful examination of the "Ring" and other exercises which appear in this work. Are they not completely adapted to the obvious necessities of our bodies?

MUSIC WITH GYMNASTICS.

A party may dance without music. I have seen it done. But the exercise is a little dull.

Exercises with the upper extremities are as much improved by music as those with the lower extremities. Indeed with the former there is much more need of music, as the arms make no noise, such as might secure concert in exercises with the lower extremities.

A small drum, costing perhaps $5, which may be used as a bass drum, with one beating stick, with

2

which any one may keep time, is, I suppose, the sort of music most classes in gymnastics will use at first. And it has advantages. While it is less pleasing than some other instruments, it secures more perfect concert than any other.

The violin and piano are excellent, but on some accounts the hand-organ is the best of all.

Feeble and apathetic people, who have little courage to undertake gymnastic training, accomplish wonders under the inspiration of music. I believe five times as much muscle can be coaxed out, under this delightful stimulus, as without it.

THE GYMNASIUM.

The gymnasium must not be cold, but should be well ventilated. The best plan is to raise it to 65 or 68, and when the class begins, drop the upper sash of the windows, raising them again when the teacher announces a period of rest.

It is a common mistake to suppose that the gymnast should exercise in a cold room until he is warm. It is not difficult to accomplish this, but cold air is unfavorable to the development of muscle. My own rule is to make the hall as warm as for a lecture, and then open the windows freely during the exercise.

The floor of the gymnasium should be marked as shown in the cut. The lines must be about fifty-five inches apart, both lengthwise and crosswise of the room. The feet must have exactly the relations exhibited in the cut. A large piece of tin, cut out in the shape of a pair of feet, and laid on the floor at the right points, may be used with a stencil brush, to make the marks. The painters will furnish a black paint which contains no oil. It is very little trouble to mark a floor in this way.

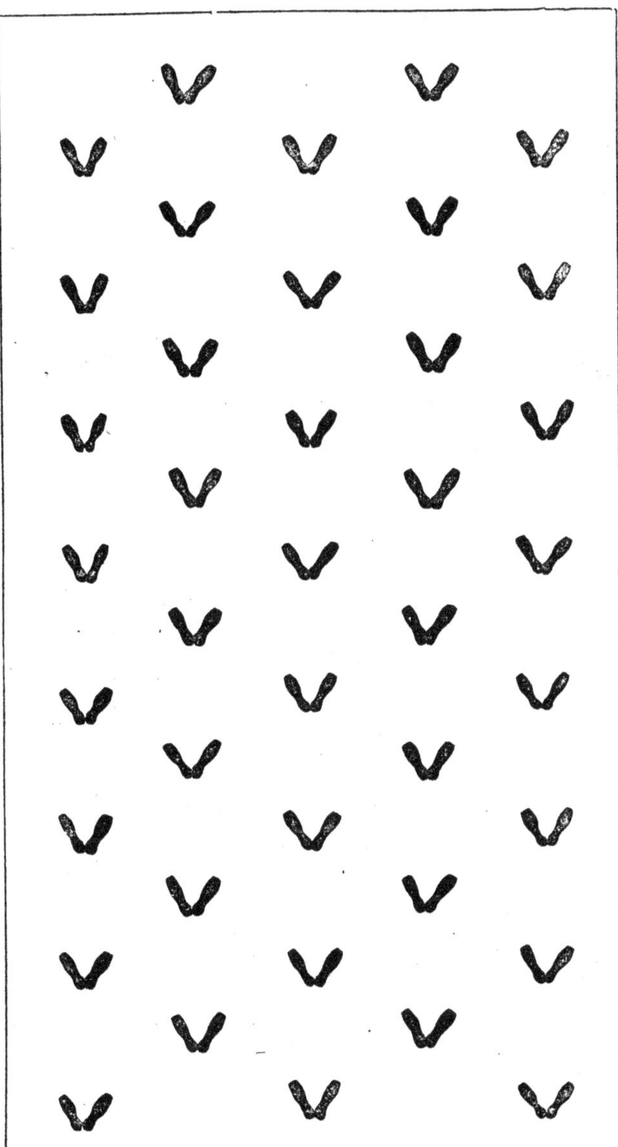

With a floor thus marked, you have to make no explanations, either in regard to the position of each pupil on the floor, or the attitude of the feet, and you are sure to avoid all accidents.

It is very difficult to keep the floor of a gymnasium sufficiently clean, but it is better to refrain from gymnastic training altogether, than to expose the lungs of the pupil to a cloud of dust. Complete gymnastics involve much foot stamping, designed to invigorate the circulation in our feet and legs, which are generally cold No feature of the exercises is more important. How shall freedom from dust be secured? In my own gymnasium, I have the floor cleansed with water three times a week. Scattering damp saw dust over the floor and sweeping it off, has been resorted to with satisfaction.

But if the floor have many cracks, they fill with dust, which the stamping will not fail to bring out. In such a case it is well to fill the cracks with wax, which, being melted, can be filled in with little difficulty. When the wax has been thoroughly cleansed from the upper surface of the boards, it will not work up from the cracks and make the boards slippery.

GYMNASTIC DRESS.

The accompanying cuts present good illustrations of the costume worn during the performance of the New Gymnastics. The most essential feature of the dress is perfect liberty about the waist and shoulders. The female costume may be never so short, if the waist or shoulders be trammelled, the exertions will serve no good purpose. If the arms can be thrust perpendicularly upward without drawing a quarter of an ounce on the dress, the most vital point has been secured.

It is made very loose about the waist and shoulders, worn without hoops, but with a thin skirt as near the color of the dress as possible, and only stiff enough to keep the outside skirt from hanging closely to the legs. This skirt should be fastened to the belt of the dress so that it will not hang below the dress when the arms are raised.

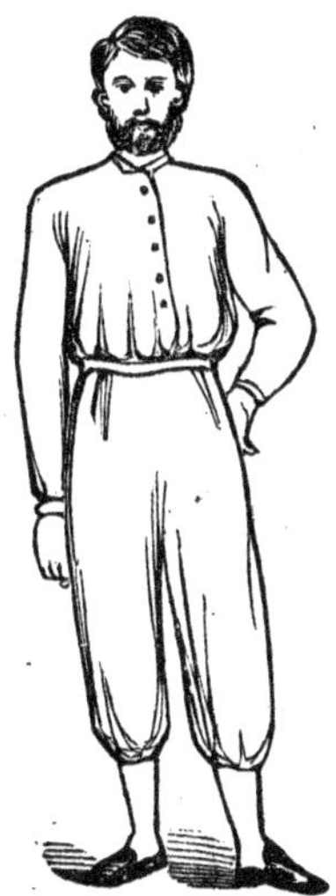

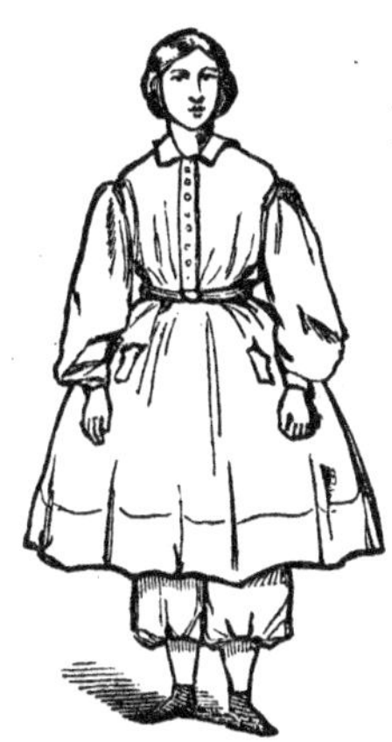

The present style of Garibaldi waist is very beautiful. It is particularly appropriate for gymnastics, as it allows the freest action of the arms and shoulders. But to permit this waist to fall over the belt, which is its peculiar feature, the belt is usually made tight enough to keep it in its position. This is wrong. Buttons should be placed on the inside of the belt, the same as on gentlemen's pants for suspenders, and the same kind of suspenders should be worn. In this way the belt may be very loose, and yet being supported over the shoulders, it will remain in its proper position.

It will be observed the gentlemen's dress has no belt. The jacket is buttoned to the pants, as is the fashion with small boys. The tailor will easily manage to conceal the buttons. The dress about the shoulders should be *very loose*. The pants must be loose, and may be fastened at the knee, as in the Zouave dress, or worn down to the ankle.

At all seasons of the year the material should be flannel.

The shoe I am in the habit of wearing is low quartered, fastened with a strong buckle, and the bottom is covered with a layer of rubber. In many of the difficult feats the foot is apt to slip, unless the rubber is added.

A majority of my pupils simply remove their coats and exercise in the street dress, but the garb I have described, has signal advantages.

BAG EXERCISES.

The use of small bags filled with beans, for gymnastic exercise, was suggested to my mind six years since, while attempting to devise a series of games with large rubber balls. Throwing and catching objects in certain ways, requiring skill and presence of mind, affords not only good exercise of the muscles of the arms and upper half of the body, but cultivates a quickness of eye and coolness of nerve very desirable. Appreciating this, I employed large rubber balls, but was constantly annoyed at the irregularities resulting from the difficulty in catching them. When the balls were but partially inflated, it was observed the hand could better seize them. This at length suggested the bean bags. Six years' use of these bags has resulted in the adoption of the following, as the best size and shape:

The material is a strong bed-ticking. Bags for young children should be, before sewing, seven inches square; for ladies, nine inches; for ladies and gentlemen exercising together, ten inches; for gentlemen alone, twelve inches. Sew them with strong linen or silk thread, doubled, nearly three quarters of an inch from the edge, leaving a small opening at one corner to pour in the beans. Fill the bags three quarters full, and they are ready for use. If used daily, once in two weeks they should be emptied and washed. To allow them to be played with after they are soiled, is pretty sure to furnish much dust for the lungs of the players, beside soiling the hands and clothes. There cannot be too much care exercised in regard to this point of cleanliness. Before the beans are used the first time, they should be rinsed with water until it runs from them quite clean, when they must be dried; and every month or two afterwards this cleansing should be repeated.

The dirty carelessness with which these bag exercises are generally managed, makes them a positive nuisance.

Premising this indispensable preparation and care of the bags, I shall now proceed to give those exercises which I have found best adapted to schools and the gymnasium.

Fig. 1, represents a series of hoops lashed between

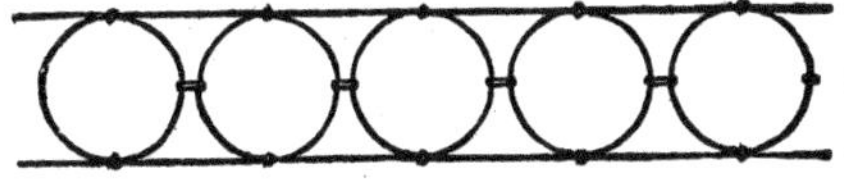

two strong ropes, and stretched across the room,

the ropes fastened on one side of the room into staples, and on the other running through pulleys. By these means the ropes may be drawn very taut. It is well to fasten the staples and pulleys into slides, that the altitude of the hoops may be altered, for persons of different ages.

Nearly all the exercises with bags are greatly improved by throwing them through the hoops. It will be observed the cuts represent the players as throwing the bags quite high. This has reference to the hoops. But the bags may be thrown between the players without the hoops.

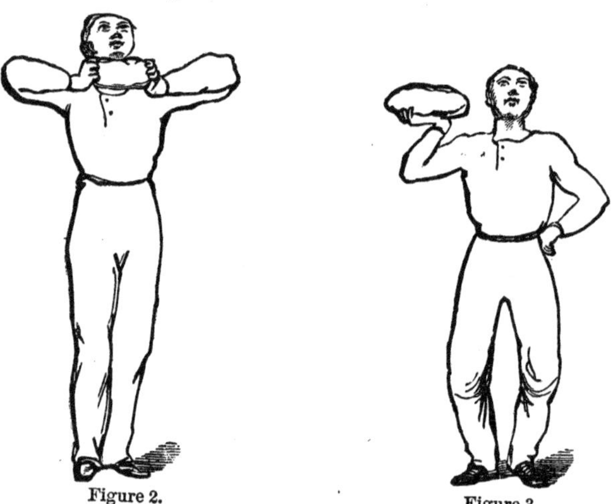

Figure 2. Figure 3.

No. 1. Arrange yourselves in two classes. Classes face each other, six feet apart. Members of one class will each have a bag. The other class will have no bags. Each person will play with the one standing exactly opposite. Hold the bags under your chins. (*Fig.* 2.) When I give the word, each couple is to throw its bag backward and forward ten times, counting both ways. At the beginning of this and the following exercises, the leader will announce how many times the bag is to be thrown.

Each couple will play as rapidly as possible, and as each finishes, the two players will hold up their hands, and cry out the number in a loud voice. Now ready! *One*, *two*, THREE!! The bag is always to be thrown from the chest, never to be tossed from the lap.

No. 2. Same as the last, except the bag is thrown and caught with the right hand. The position is well shown in *Fig*. 3.

No. 3. Same as the last, but with the left hand. When the right hand throws, the partner's right hand must catch, and so with the left.

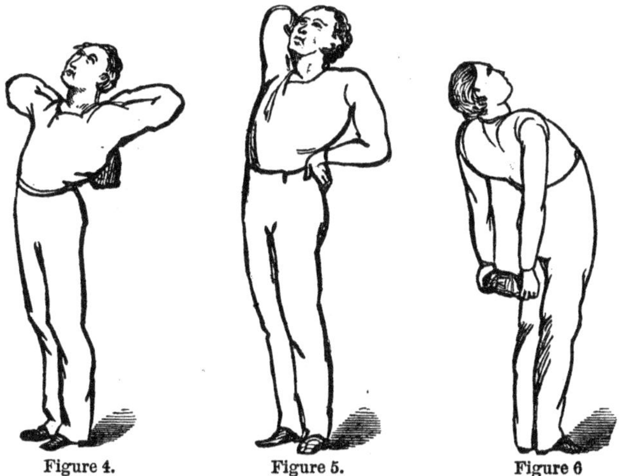

Figure 4. Figure 5. Figure 6

No. 4. In this one, the bag is thrown with both hands, from the position seen in *Fig*. 4.

No. 5. Same as the last, except the bag is thrown with the right hand, as shown in *Fig*. 5. The unoccupied hand in this and all other single-handed bag exercises is to be held on the corresponding side, with the arm akimbo.

No. 6. Same as the last, except with the left hand.

No. 7. The bag is to be thrown over the head from the position seen in *Fig.* 6.

No. 8. To be thrown from the position seen in *Fig.* 7, with the right hand. The one who catches must receive it, while the left hand grasps the arm in the same way.

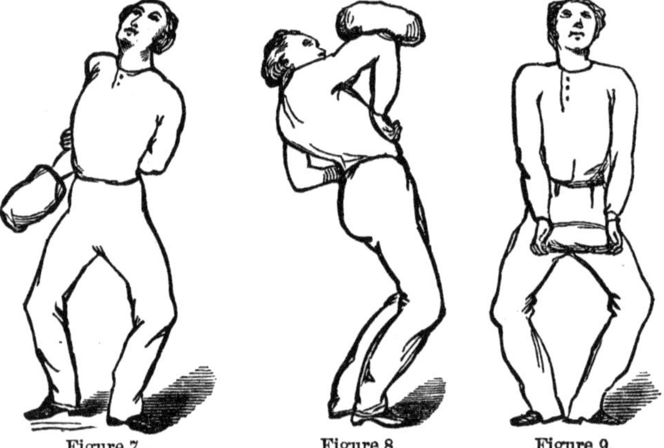

Figure 7. Figure 8. Figure 9.

No. 9. Same as the last, only using the left hand.

No. 10. Standing with your right side toward your partner, hold the bag on the point of the elbow, being sure to keep the fore-arm vertical; (*Fig.* 8) throw from this position the number of times announced by the leader. To be caught in the hands.

No. 11. Same as the last, except the left side is turned, and the bag is thrown from the left elbow.

No. 12. Hold the bag as represented in *Fig.* 9, and toss to your partner. He will of course return it in the same manner to you, and thus it will be tossed backward and forward the number of times indicated by the leader. As in all the other exercises thus far given, each couple upon reaching the indicated number, will hold up their hands and cry out that number in a loud voice.

No. 13. Turning your right side to your partner, throw from the position represented in *Fig*. 10. Your partner catches the bag, standing in the same attitude.

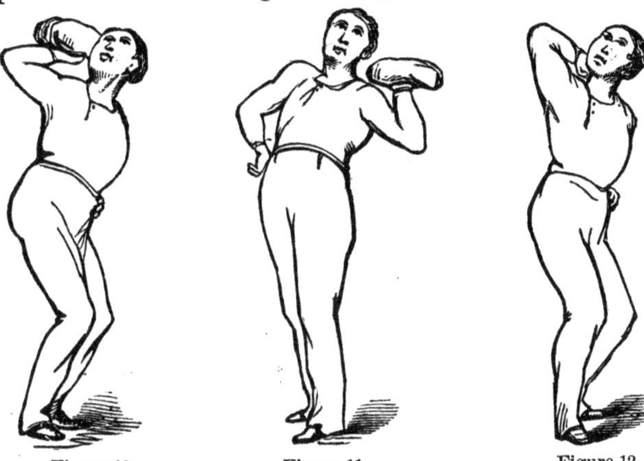

Figure 10. Figure 11. Figure 12.

No. 14. Same as the last, except you turn your left side to your partner, and throw with the left hand, either without bending the knees, as seen in *Fig*. 11, or bending them, as seen in *Fig*. 10.

No. 15. Again turn your right side to your partner, and throw the bag from the position seen in *Fig*. 12.

No. 16. Same as the last, except turning the left side, you throw with the left hand.

No. 17. Turn your back to your partner, and bend backwards, so that you can see him. He bends back, so that he may see you, and then you throw the bag to him as represented in *Fig*. 13. Always cry *ready!*

that he may not be kept waiting too long in an uncomfortable position.

No. 18. Face your partner, and throw from the position represented in *Fig.* 14, holding the bag on the back of the hand.

No. 19. Same as the last, except the left hand is employed.

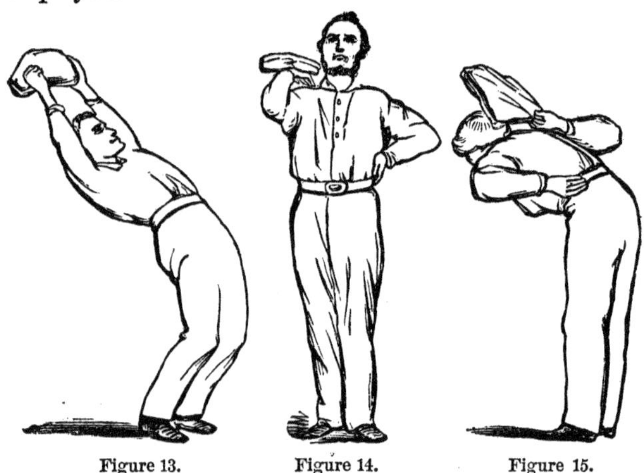

Figure 13. Figure 14. Figure 15.

No. 20. Face your partner, and throw the bag around the back and over the opposite shoulder, as shown in *Fig.* 15.

No. 21. Same as the last, except you use the other hand.

No. 22. Each couple having ten bags; you throw to your partner, and he catches as many as he can hold, folding his arms. (*Fig.* 16.) This one will not ordinarily be played in class, as the number of bags will scarcely be sufficient.

No. 23. The two classes will stand as represented in *Fig.* 17. Place ten bags on a chair or box at the feet of the first player of each class. The leader gives the word, *one*, *two*, *three!* and the two classes compete in passing the bags over their heads backwards, to the foot of the class, when they whirl round and immediately pass them back. The class which has the entire ten on the chair or box at its head, first, counts one in the game. It is usual to make the game three, five, or ten.

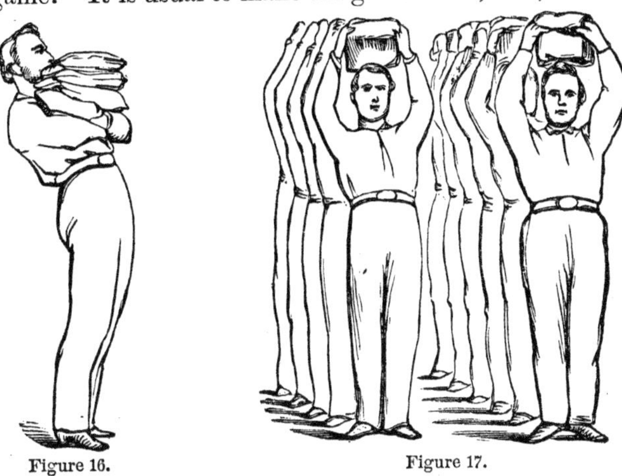

Figure 16. Figure 17.

No. 24. Let the two classes face each other again, and pass the bags as in the last, except that they are carried along in front and as high as the chest, being careful not to stoop forward.

No. 25. Let the bags be all placed at the head of one of the classes. We will call this class No. 1; the other class No. 2. The first player in class No. 1, throws a bag to the first player in class No. 2, who throws it back to the second player in class No. 1, who throws it back to the second player in class No. 2, who, in turn, throws it to the third player in class No. 1, and so on, working it down to the foot of the class.

But one bag is not allowed to make the trip alone; all follow, one after another, in rapid succession.

In this game, the bags are all thrown from the chest with both hands, as represented some pages back, in No. 1, of the bag exercises.

No. 26. The whole company may now be divided into trios, each trio playing with three bags, as represented in *Fig.* 18. Each one throws the bag to the player at his right hand, and at the same time catches the bag thrown from the player at his left.

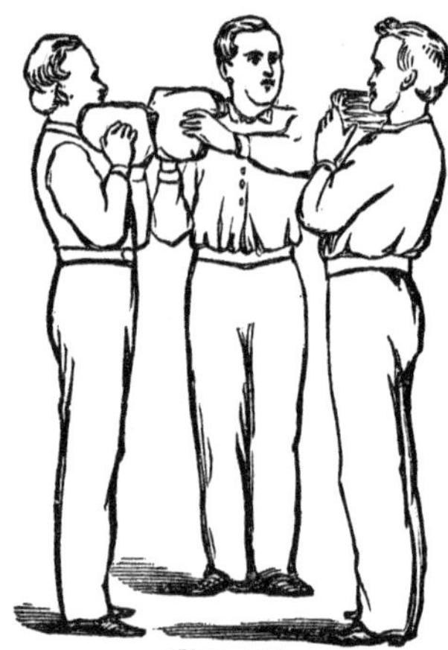

Figure 18.

To secure the proper distance between the players for this game, they should take each other by the hands, and pulling hard, they will have the right positions. Each player must look constantly at the one from whom he receives the bags, and never for a moment at the one to whom he throws. If they forget this rule, the bags will soon fall to the floor.

No. 27. Same as the last, except the bags are passed the opposite way.

No. 28. The company is again divided into couples, and each couple plays with two, three, four, or more bags. A throws a bag with his right hand to B, who catches it with his left hand, and immediately changing it to his right, throws it back to A, who catches it with his left, and who changing it to his right, throws it back again to B. (*Fig.* 19.) Two, three, four, or five bags can be made to perform this circle between two players at the same time.

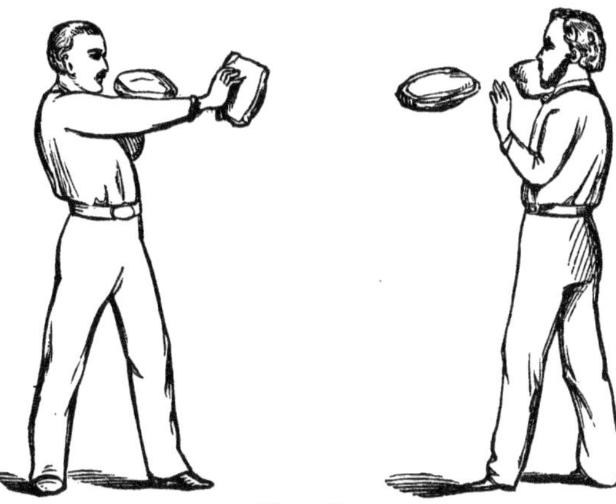

Figure 19.

The bags, in this as in all the other bag exercises, except one, should be thrown and not tossed.

No. 29. Same as the last, except the bags are thrown with the left and caught with the right hand.

No. 30. Now the players will stand in two classes again, the classes to be six feet apart, and the players in each party to be six feet from each other. Place six bags on a chair at the head of each class. Upon the word *one*, *two*, THREE ! the first player in each class seizes a bag and runs with it to the second player, who carries it to the third, who in turn rushes to the fourth, and so on to the foot of the class. But one bag is not allowed to make the journey alone. One at a time, the whole six are hurried onward. Instantly and without any signal they are sent back to the head of the class in the same order. The class which has its six bags on the chair at the head of the class first, counts one in the game.

EXERCISES WITH RINGS.

This series of exercises is entirely new, and beyond all comparison, the best ever devised. Physiologists and Gymnasts have everywhere bestowed upon it the most unqualified commendation. Indeed it is difficult to conceive any other possible series so complete in a physiological point of view, and so happily adapted to family, school, and general use.

If a man were as strong as Sampson, he would find in the use of these rings, with another man of equal strength, the fullest opportunity to exert his utmost strength; while the frailest child, engaged with one of equal strength, would never be injured.

There is not a muscle in the entire body which may not be brought into direct play through the medium of the rings. And if one particular muscle, or set of muscles is especially deficient or weak, the exercise may be concentrated upon that muscle or set of muscles.

Wherever these rings are introduced they will obtain the highest favor and awaken the most earnest enthusiasm.

The ring is generally turned from cherry wood, and when finished measures six inches in diameter, while the body is one inch thick. It should be highly polished, especially on the inner part. *Fig.* 1 gives a good idea of the ring.

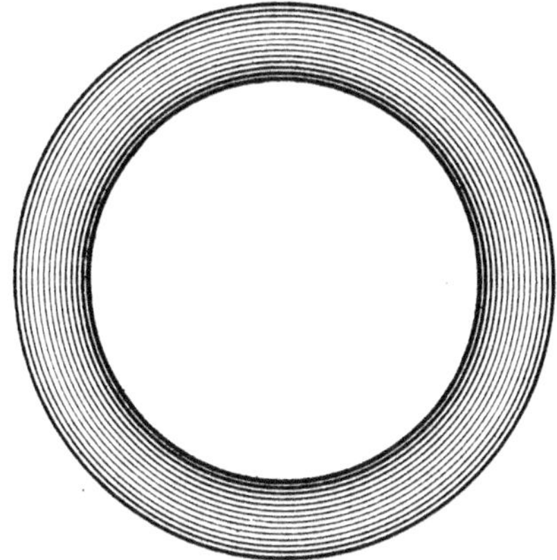

Figure 1.

No. 1. Standing in the position represented in *Fig.* 2, the end of the right toe against the right toe of your partner, the toes meeting on a straight line drawn through the entire hall, on which all the players stand, and placing the left foot at right angles with the right foot, as seen in the figure; pull hard and twist the right arm hard from right to left and left to right ten times, keeping time to the music.

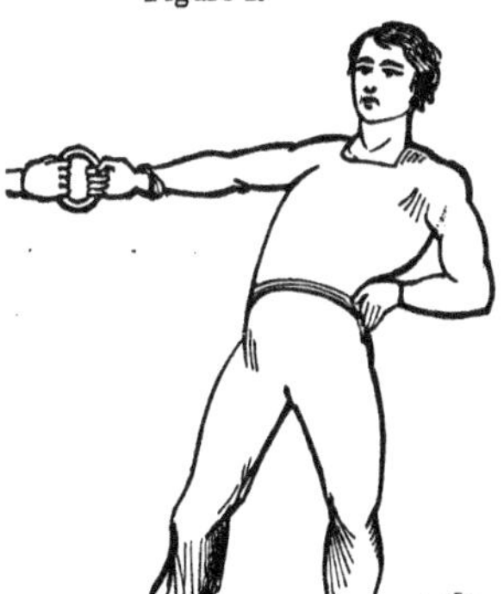

Figure 2.

Be careful in this, as in all other exercises with the ring to draw the shoulders well back and keep the head erect.

No. 2. Same as the last, but using the left hand with the left foot forward.

No. 3. Join both hands with two rings, and place the right toe against your partner's right toe as in No. 1, being sure to keep the foot which is behind at right angles with the one in front, (which I may say here, is to be looked after with much care through this whole series, whenever it is possible,) then pull hard, ten times, and twist the arms, keeping time to the music.

No. 4. Exactly the same as the last, but with the left foot forward.

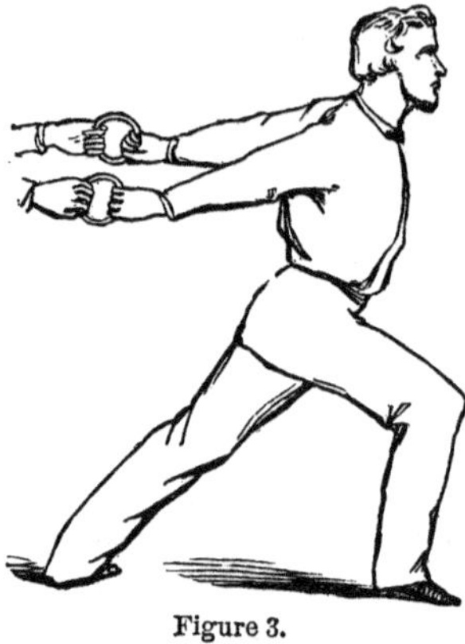
Figure 3.

No. 5. Without letting go the rings, turn back to back, place the outside of your left foot against the same of your partner, in the same way you would push against the wall of the room, and pulling hard in the position represented in *Fig.* 3, twist hard ten times, keeping time to the music.

No. 6. Same as the last, but with the right foot behind.

No. 7. Turn face to face, raise the hands as high as you can over the head, and standing about two feet and a half apart, bring the rings down to the floor without bending the knees, as represented in *Fig.* 4, ten times, and all the following exercises ten times. In the performance of this you must not bend the elbows, which you can avoid doing by carrying the rings outward at each side. (In the ring exercises, when your pupils, standing their faces toward each other, turn their backs, see that they do not let go the rings.)

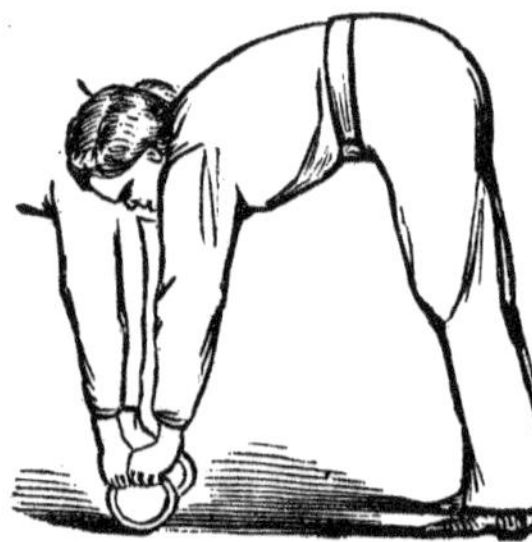
Figure 4.

No. 8. Standing as in the last exercise, but only

two feet apart, place the rings in the position seen in *Fig*. 5. Now as the arms on one side rise, the arms on the other side fall, keeping time to the music. Be careful not to bend the arms at the elbows, which of course can be prevented in this as in many other exercises, by carrying the hands outward at the side. In this exercise a good deal of force should be used, so that when the ring is carried up on one side, it goes far beyond the perpendicular line, the bodies of the players bending freely.

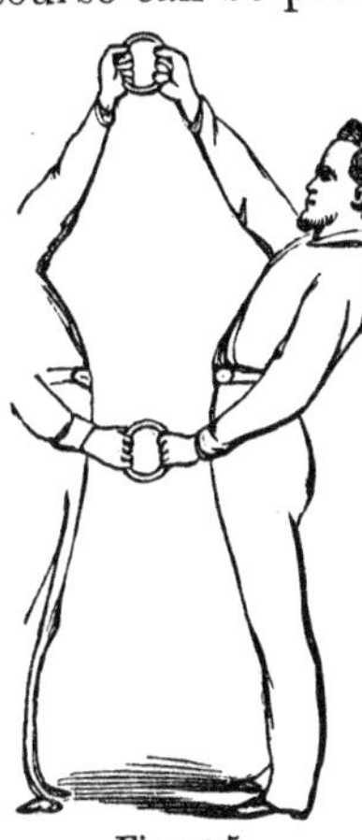
Figure 5.

No. 9. Same as the last, except the two rings go up and down simultaneously.

No. 10. Standing as in the last two exercises, the hands hanging down as low as may be, and keeping them in the same relation to each other, swing them from side to side as far as you can.

No. 11. Same as the last, except that instead of wisnging the hands from side to side, they make a complete circle, being carried over the head as well as down between the bodies of the players.

No. 12. Same as the last, except the circle is made the opposite way.

No. 13. Back to back, as seen in *Fig*. 6, thrust the rings up with great force, each player keeping his two arms exactly parallel.

No. 14. From the same position seen in *Fig*. 6, thrust the rings out sidewise, as in all the other exercises, ten times.

No. 15. Same as the last, except the rings are thrust downward by the hips.

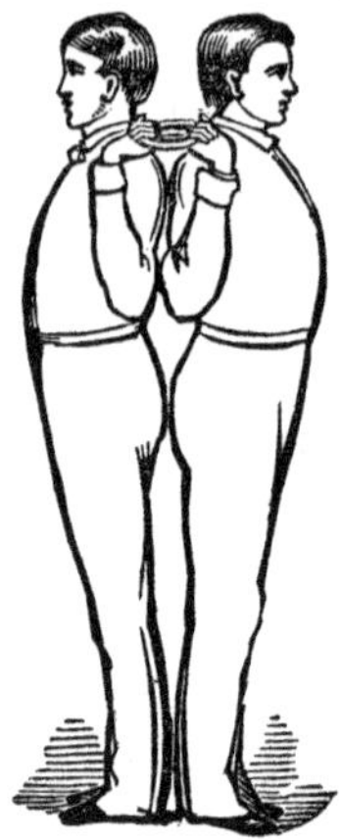

Figure 6.

No. 16. The last three, consecutively, ten times.

No. 17. Take the position seen in *Fig.* 7; your partner the same. The inside of your left foot to the inside of his left. Draw your left hand as far back past your left side as possible, dragging your partner's right hand after it. At the same time he has done the same thing with his left. Do the same with your right hands. And so continue to alternate. Do this strongly, pushing your hand past your partner's side as far as possible, at the same time pulling his hand as far past yours as possible.

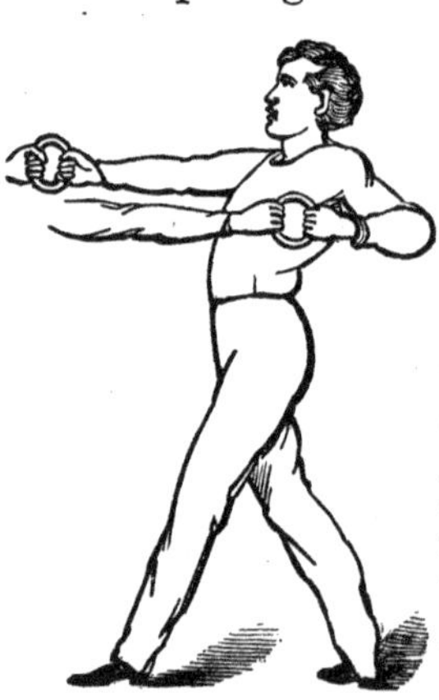

Figure 7.

No. 18. Same as the last, except the right foot is forward. Be sure in this as in all others, that your two feet are at right angles.

No. 19. Same as the last two, except the feet go with the hands. When you thrust your right hand forward, the right foot goes forward too. When the left hand goes forward, the left foot goes with it.

If this be well done, the feet and hands making long sweeps to the music, it not only presents a fine, animated appearance to the spectators, but brings all the muscles of the body and limbs into fine play.

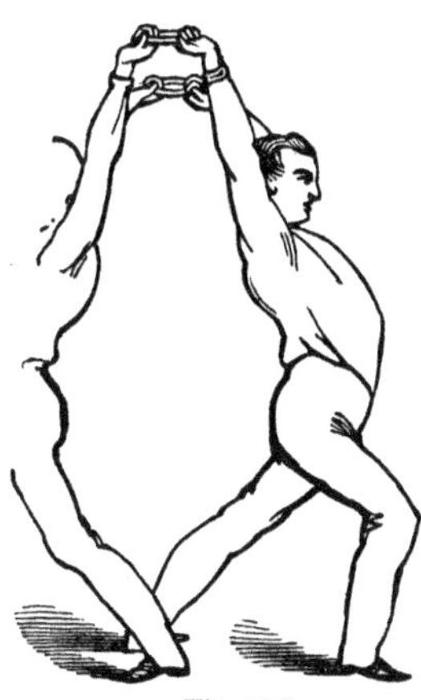

Figure 8.

No. 20. Back to back, touching each other's heels. Each lunge out with the right foot in the direction the toe points, the feet being at right angles, and raise the hands over the head so they touch, thus reaching the position seen in *Fig*. 8. Now back, heels together, arms at the side, lunge out with the left feet in the same way, and thus alternate, keeping time to the music.

No. 21. Standing as represented in *Fig*. 9, your partner the same, with the inside of his left foot to the inside of your left foot, and holding the rings as shown in the figure, push them vigorously toward your partner, simultaneously thrusting them past his body as far as possible. He pushes them back in the same manner, and so on.

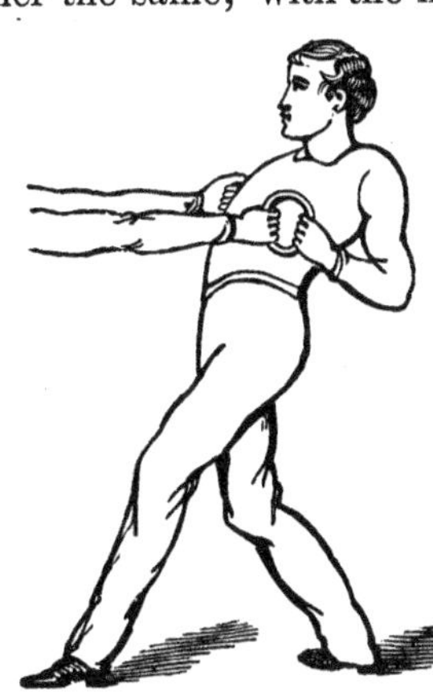

Figure 9.

No. 22. Same as the last, except the right foot is pushed forward, instead of the left.

No. 23. Stand back to back, heels all together; both step out sidewise in the same direction as far as you can reach, and at the same instant raise the hands on the same side as high as you can, then returning to the upright position, hands by your sides, charge out at the other side in a similar manner. When this has been done both ways, as in every other exercise, ten times; the leader cries "alternately," and you continue to charge sideways as before, only in opposite directions as represented in *Fig.* 10.

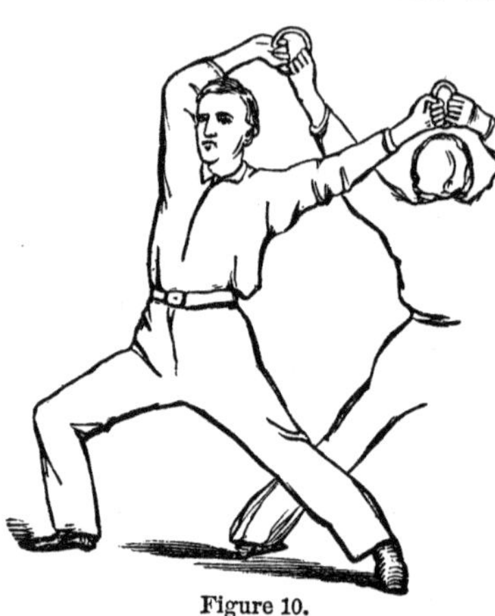

Figure 10.

No. 24. Standing face to face, two feet apart, charge sideways as in the last exercise, and as seen in *Fig.* 11. In alternation with this, charge the opposite way. After the regular number of times, the teacher cries "alternately," and you charge out sideways with your right feet in opposite ways, as seen in *Fig.* 12; alternate with the left feet.

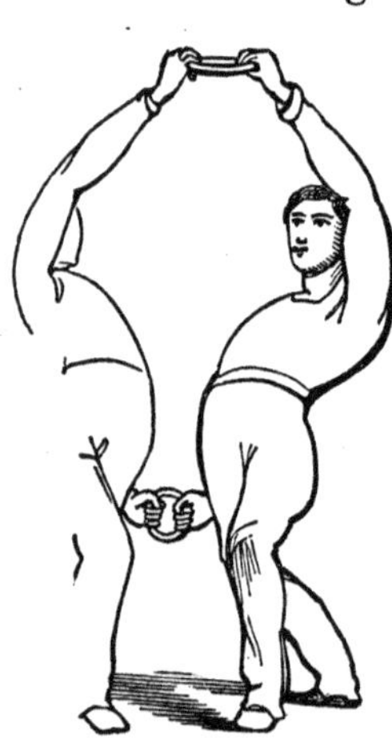

Figure 11.

No. 25. Standing back to back, charge, your faces both in one direction, with bodies fronting the same, as shown in *Fig.* 13. When the teacher cries "*change!*" you must change sides with each other, still facing in the same direction. Keep time to the music with your feet, when changing sides, and as soon as you make the change, go on with the charging, using of course, the other hands and feet.

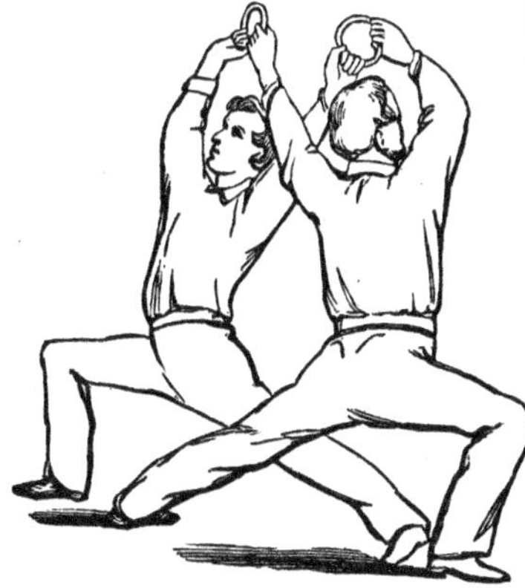

Figure 12.

No. 26. Joining only with your right hands, and standing apart far enough to make the arms straight and horizontal between you, charge as seen in *Fig.* 14; the left hand and foot the same.

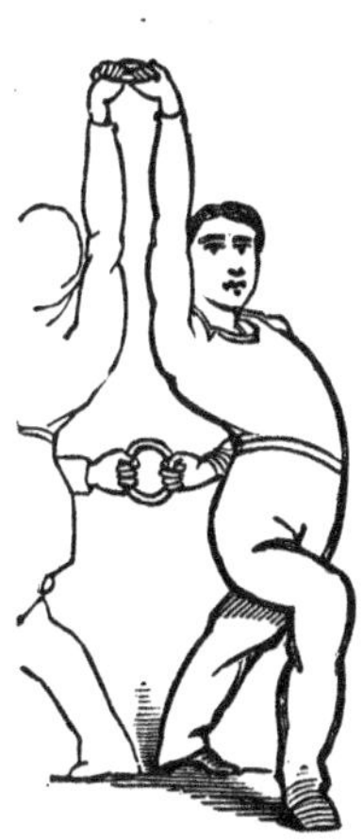

Figure 13.

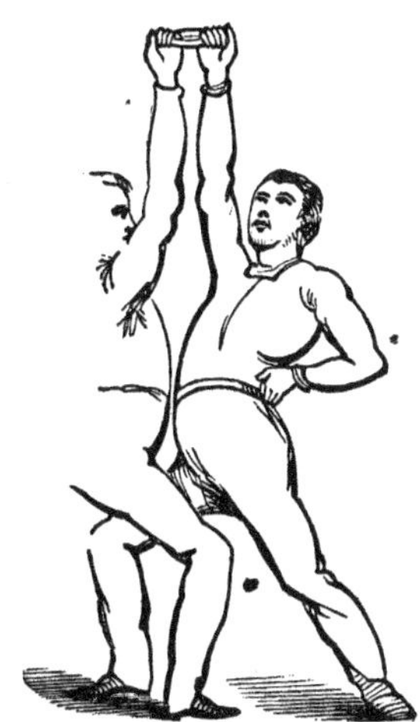

Figure 14.

No. 27. Joining with both hands, charge right and

left alternately, each time, as represented in *Fig.* 14.

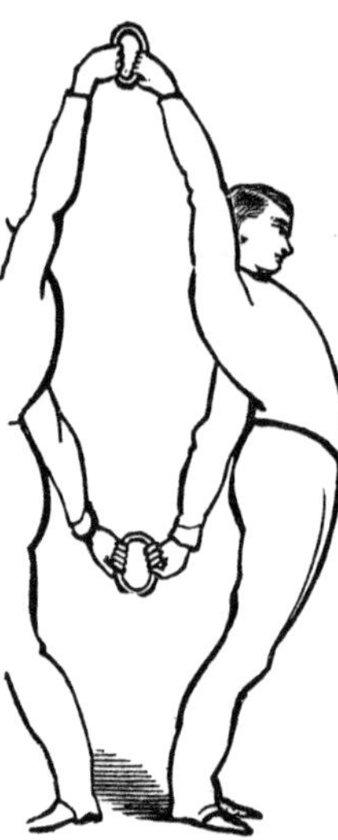
Figure 15.

No. 28. Stand, each with his own heels together, as seen in *Fig.* 15, and perform the exercise exhibited in the figure. As the hands on one side go up, the hands on the other go down. So alternate the regular number of times, when you will do the same simultaneously, the hands on both sides rising and falling together.

No. 29. Standing as seen in *Fig.* 16, except that the inside of the right foot should be exhibited as pressing against the inside of your partner's right foot, you draw back from each other as far as you can, and then come up, touching each other's chests, all without bending the elbows.

No. 30. Same, with the left foot forward.

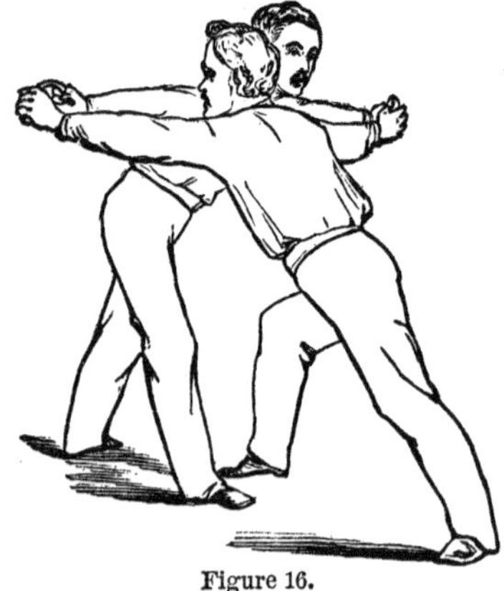
Figure 16.

No. 31. Standing as seen in *Fig.* 17, draw far away from each other, keeping the arms precisely horizontal. Immediately approaching each other again, touch the shoulders as in the figure, and so continue ten times, keeping time to the music.

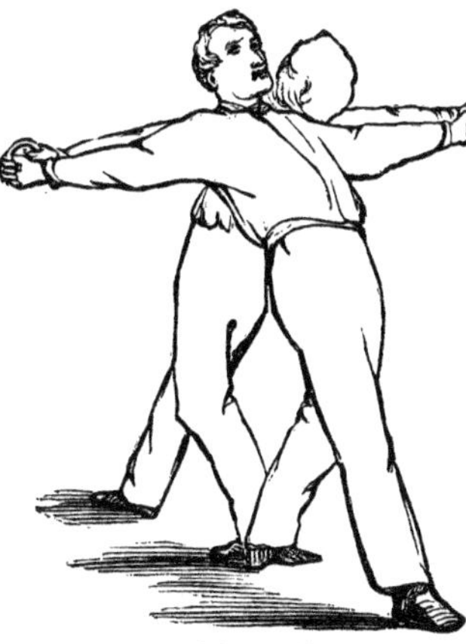

Figure 17.

No. 32. Same as the last, with the feet changed.

No. 33. Standing face to face, raise the hands on one side as in *Fig.* 18. As these hands are brought down to the side, raise those on the other side in like manner, and so alternate ten times.

No. 34. Back to back, and raise the arms on one side as in *Fig.* 18, but carry the hands completely over the heads and down on the other side of the body. Alternate with the arms on the other side, ten times.

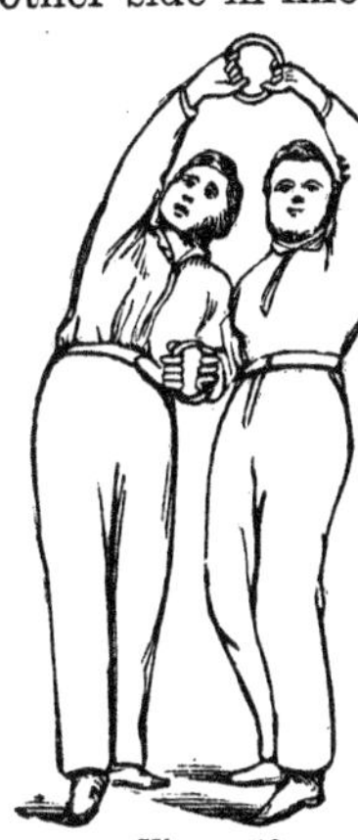

Figure 18.

No. 35. Carry the hands all over together, as seen in *Fig.* 19. Change thus from side to side, twenty times, always keeping time to the music.

No. 36. Turn face to face, and now back to back, and again face to face, and so continue to change, alternating the sides toward which you turn.

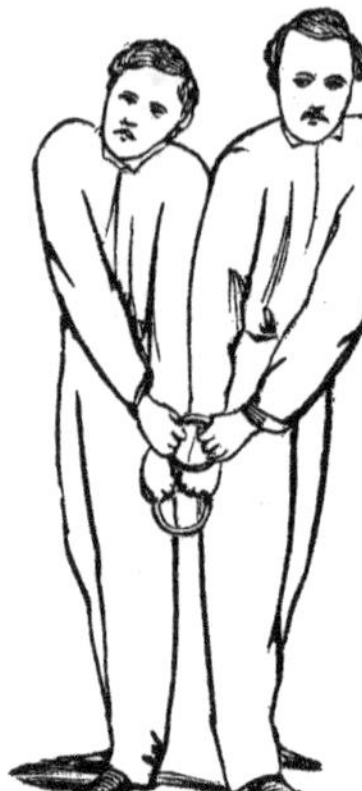
Figure 19.

No. 37. Perform the exercise seen in *Fig.* 20, being sure that you draw the arm of your partner directly into your axilla or arm-pit. After alternating twenty times, then draw the arms back and forth simultaneously, ten times.

No. 38. Join right hands with your partner with one ring, and stand apart so that your arms are straight and horizontal. Advance your right foot two feet, keeping the two feet at a right angle. Now push your chests as near together as you can, without bending your knees or elbows, as seen in *Fig.* 21. Now drawing the arms back to the horizontal on the next beat of the music, carry the hands down as low as possible without bending knees or elbows on the next beat. Now back to the horizontal, and then up as high as possible, and so continue ten times.

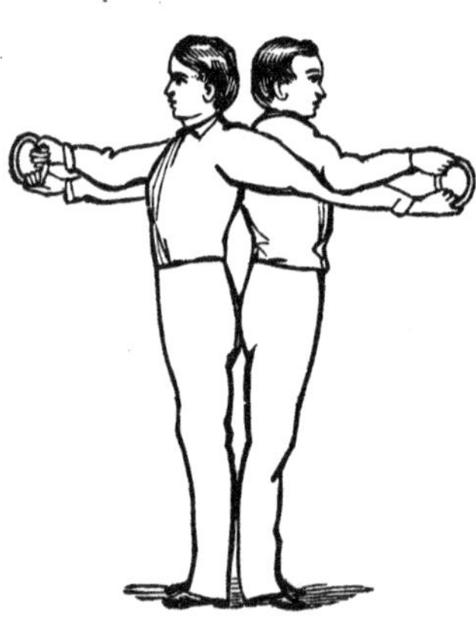
Figure 20.

No. 39. Same with the left hands, the left foot being pushed forward.

No. 40. Join the right hands again, holding them in the horizontal position.

Now push them sidewise as far as possible without bending knees or elbows. On the next beat bring the arms back to the straight line between you, and now carry them sidewise the other way, and so continue ten times.

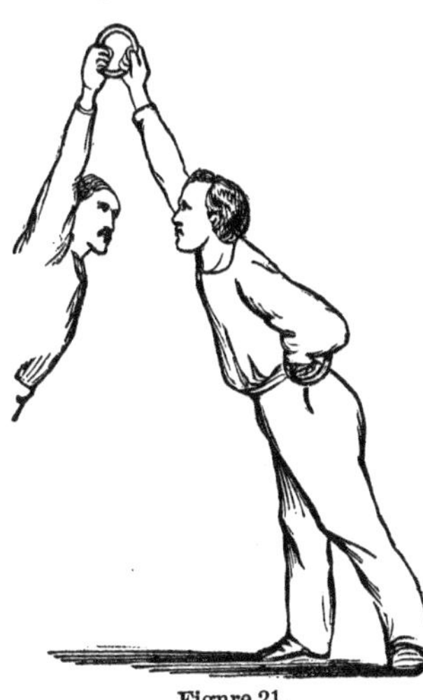
Fignre 21.

No. 41. Left hands the same.

No. 42. Join right hands again. Instead of thrusting the hands directly upward, or sidewise, carry them obliquely upward, and after bringing them back to the straight, horizontal line, carry obliquely downward, and so continue ten times, being careful not to bend knees or elbows.

No. 43. Still use the right hands, and carry them obliquely upward the other way, and downward the other way.

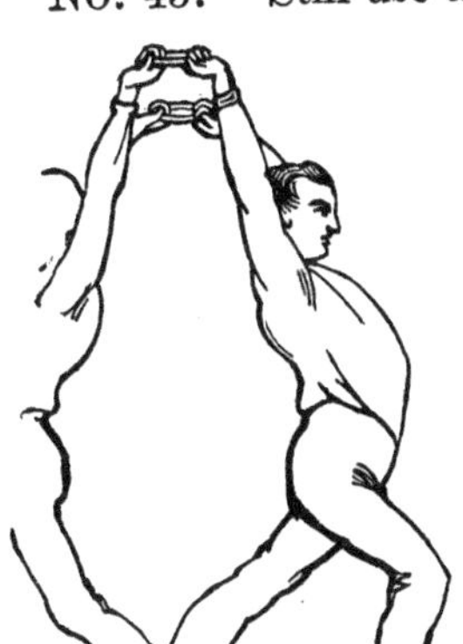
Figure 22.

Nos. 44 and 45. Same with the left hands.

No. 46. Back to back, and place the outside of the left foot against the outside of your partner's left foot. Right foot well forward. Now raise the hands over the head as seen in *Fig*. 22, (I see the artist has not placed the outsides of the left feet against each other, as he should have done) and draw away from each other, bending the knee of the leg which is pushed forward, and thus sink down somewhat. As you come back, touch your shoulders against those of your partner, and thus repeat ten times.

No. 47. Same, with a change of feet.

In the last two exercises, as you draw away, you must not pull on the rings a single ounce. If this be forgotten your backs may be hurt.

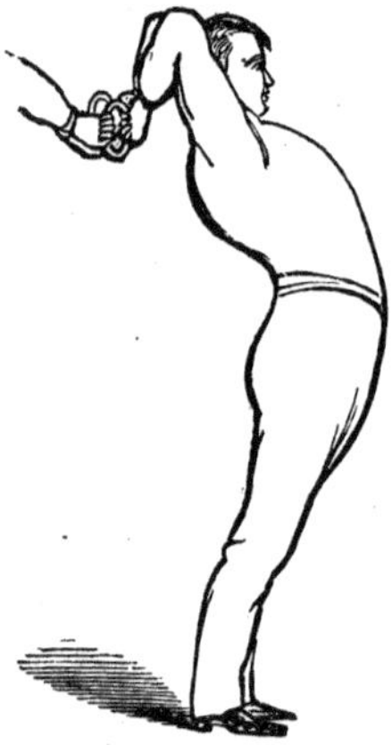

No. 48. Face to face, join the right hands, and place the tips of the right toes against each other, and the left feet at right angles two feet behind. Whirl the right hands, making as large a circle as possible without bending the elbows or knees. After whirling ten times one way, then whirl ten times the other way.

No. 49. Same with left hands.

Figure 23.

No. 50. Back to back, two feet apart, each with his own heels together; raise the hands as high as possible over the heads and bring them down as seen in *Fig.* 23, five times.

No. 51. Join the right hands, and turn your right side toward your partner, keeping the right arms straight between you. Both must now step straight forward with the right foot as far as you can reach, while the right arms are kept horizontal, as seen in *Fig.* 24.

No. 52. Face the opposite way, and use the left arms and feet in the same manner.

No. 53. Stand as shown in *Fig.* 25. Pull your arms directly forward, which of course will draw your partner's arms directly backwards. Then he draws yours backwards in like manner, and so continue ten times.

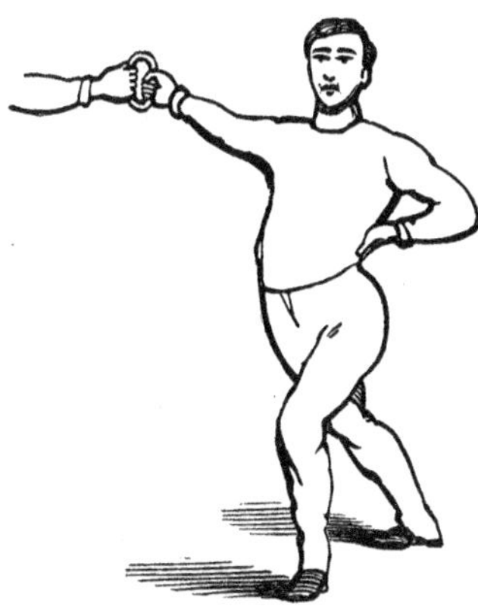

Figure 24.

No. 54. Back to back, your shoulders touching your partner. Arms perpendicular over the head. Draw your right arm directly forward. Simultaneously with this your partner does the same thing. Now the left arms the same, and so continue to alternate ten times. And last draw both of your arms forward; immediately your partner does the same, and so continue to alternate ten times.

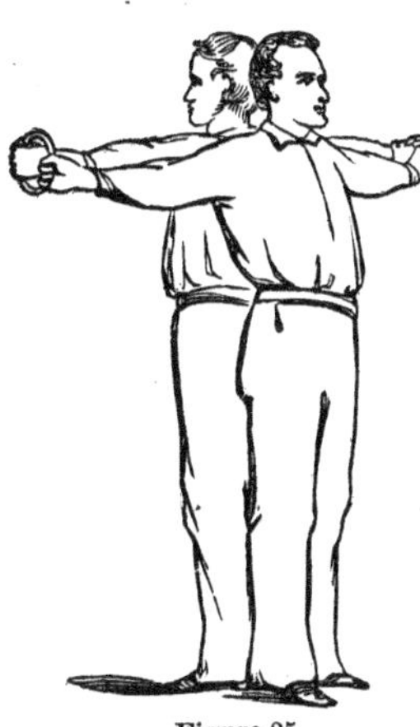

Figure 25.

These are not a quarter of the possible exercises with the rings, but after a long use of them, with much study and innumerable experiments, I believe this series gives the best variety, and is sufficiently extended. Besides, this series is admirably calculated to develope those particular muscles which are almost universally deficient in the people of the United States.

EXERCISES WITH WANDS.

A straight, smooth stick, one inch in diameter, and four feet long, (three feet for children) with round ends, is known in this Gymnasium as a "Wand," and is highly prized. It is used to cultivate flexibility, and is equally useful to persons of all ages and degrees of strength.

As a stiff, inflexible condition of the ligaments and muscles connected with the shoulders is the principal obstacle in the way of beginners, and as the wand is the best known means to remove this stiffness, it should be made prominent during the first few weeks or months of the training.

It is perhaps unnecessary to say that the symmetrical development of the upper half of the body turns entirely upon the freedom with which one can use the shoulder joint. This is sufficiently obvious, when we reflect that exercise of the body above the waist depends upon the arms, and of course upon the degree of freedom with which we can use the arms.

While it cannot be denied that certain muscles about the shoulders and chest may be developed to any degree, and the shoulders remain drooping and stiff, it is quite as undeniable that general and symmetrical development of that part of the body, (which is almost universally distorted and deficient among Americans,) can be achieved only by complete liberty about the shoulder joint, through which as a fulcrum or centre, all considerable training of the upper part of the body is derived.

I had pursued the study of Gymnastic Culture but a short time, before I saw the great importance of the wand, in a system of training adapted to the American people.

I have invented a very extended series of these exercises, some of which are here described and illustrated.

No. 1. Divide the wand into three equal parts with

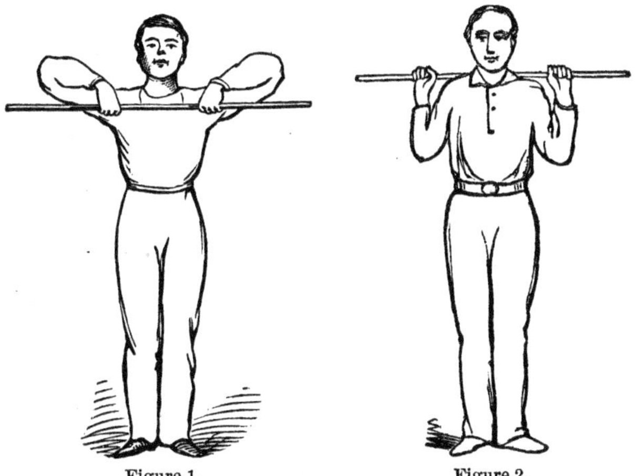

Figure 1. Figure 2.

the hands, and hold it as represented in *Fig*. 1. Thrust it downward close by the legs with much force, and again bring it up by the chin, holding the elbows high as seen in the figure, and so continue twenty times.

No. 2. From the position seen in *Fig*. 1, carry the wand directly upward as high as you can reach, and back to the chin, ten times.

No. 3. From the highest position in No. 2, bring

the wand down to the knees and back again, twenty times, *without bending the elbows.*

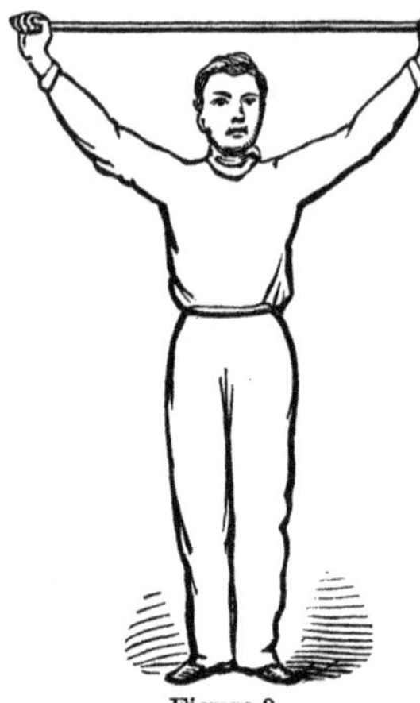
Figure 3.

No. 4. Holding the wand high over the head, bring it down on the back of the neck, ten times, as seen in *Fig.* 2.

No. 5. Same as the last, except every second time the wand is brought down to the chin, being careful that every time that the wand is carried upward, it is carried as high as possible and with much force.

No. 6. Hands over the head, but this time at the ends of the wand, as seen in *Fig.* 3, and now bring it down behind as seen in *Fig.* 4, twenty times, *being very careful not to bend the elbows.*

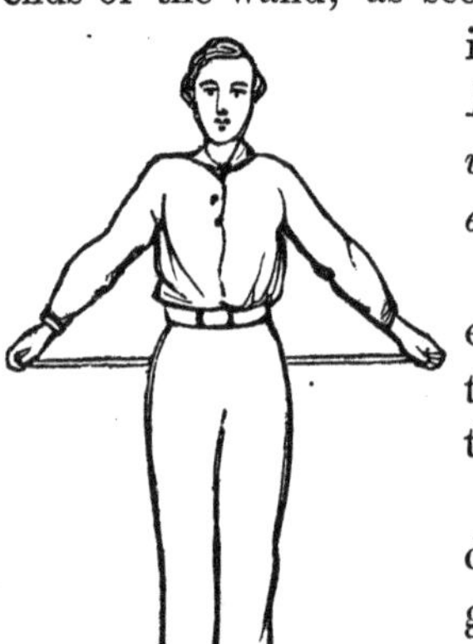
Figure 4.

No. 7. Same as the last, except that every second time the wand is brought down to the knees in front.

No. 8. Hold the wand directly over the head, hands grasping the ends, and carry it from side to side, (*Fig.* 5) being very careful not to bend the elbows, and yet the wand must come to the perpendicular on either side.

No. 9. Hold the wand directly in front and perpendicular, with the hands in the middle of it six inches apart, and the arms as nearly horizontal as possible; keeping the arms stiff, whirl the wand from side to side as far as you can.

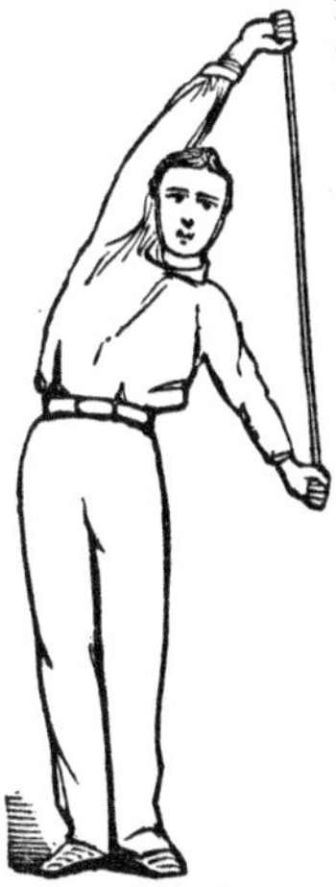

No. 10. Standing erect, heels together, put the wand out with your right hand midway between two lines, one of which runs directly forward, and the other at right angles with this, at your side; which direction we shall call diagonally forward. Let the wand rest on the floor, at a point as far removed from your feet as possible, keeping your body and the wand perpendicular, and the arm horizontal. The elbow must not be bent. Step out as seen in *Fig.* 6, the foot passing behind the wand, as seen in the figure. In doing this you must not bend the elbow, nor must you move the wand. It will be seen that the shoulders scarcely move, the motion being confined to the legs and lower part of the body. Charge thus ten times.

Figure 5.

No. 11. Same as the last, but with the left hand and foot.

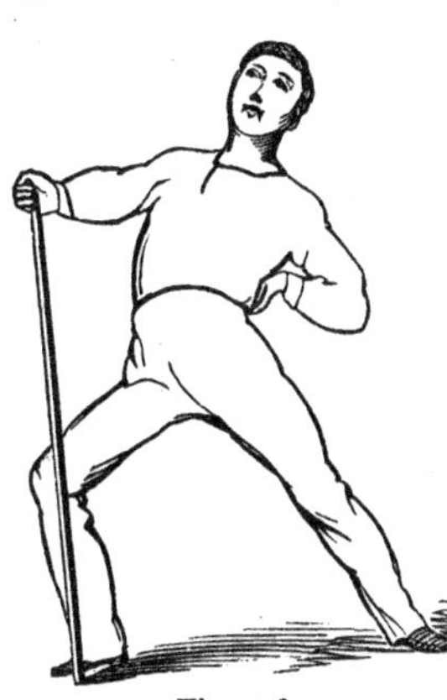

Figure 6.

No. 12. Stand erect. Carry the wand out with the left hand diagonally forward, as far as you can reach.

Step out to the wand with the left foot. Let the foot remain there. Now the body is to rise and fall as far as possible. (*Fig*. 7.) Don't bend the knee of the right leg. Keep the shoulders and head well back.

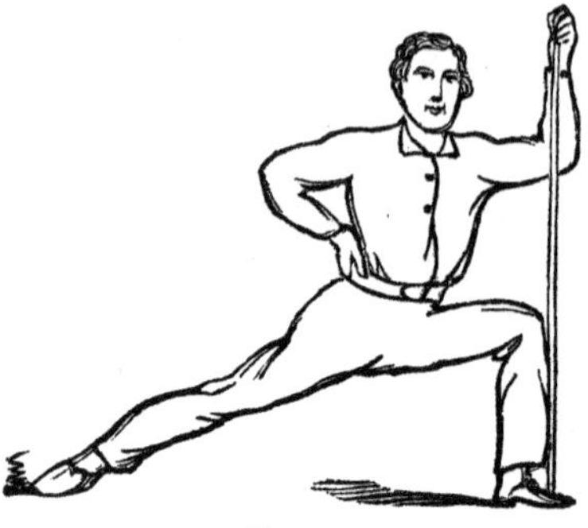

Figure 7.

No. 13. Same as the last, on the right side.

No. 14. Stand as seen in *Fig*. 8. Thrust the arms straight forward, and back again to the chest, ten times, keeping the wand all the time perpendicular.

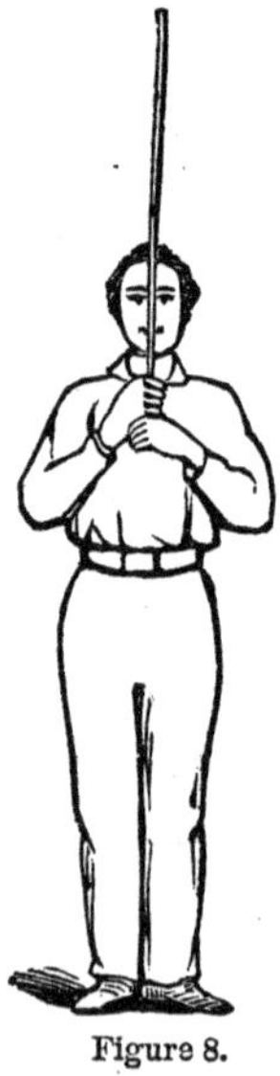

No. 15. At the conclusion of the last exercise, when the arms are thrust forward, bring the wand into the position seen in *Fig*. 9. Then carry it right back to the position in front, with the arms straight and horizontal. Now bring it down on the left side, and so continue ten times to each side.

No. 16. In concluding the last, when the arms are extended in front, bring the hands and

Figure 8.

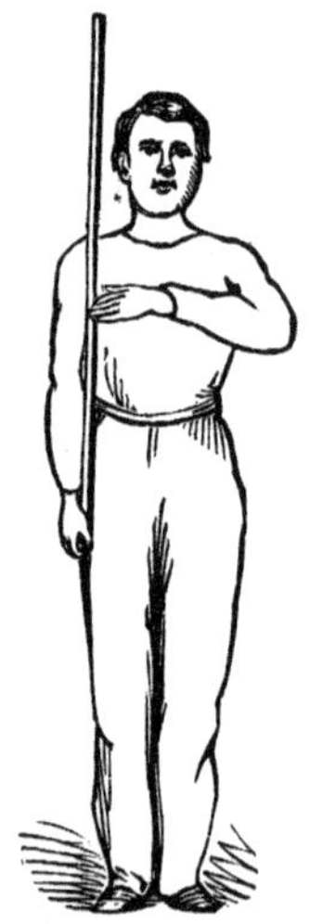

Figure 9.

wand to the position seen in *Fig*. 8. Carry it out diagonally, forward and upward on the left side, as seen in *Fig*. 10. Bring it back to the chest again, and thrust it out on the right side. Alternate twenty times.

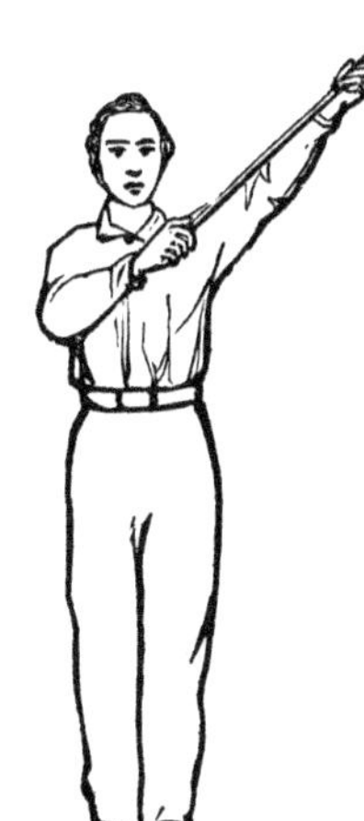

Figure 10.

No. 17. As you thrust out the wand on the right side, step out the foot in the same direction. Be sure it is neither forward or at the side, but diagonally forward. (*Fig*. 11.) Alternate between the right and left side, twenty times.

No. 18. Same as the last, except the wand goes to the right as the left foot charges to the left, and the left arm and wand to the left, while the right foot charges to the right.

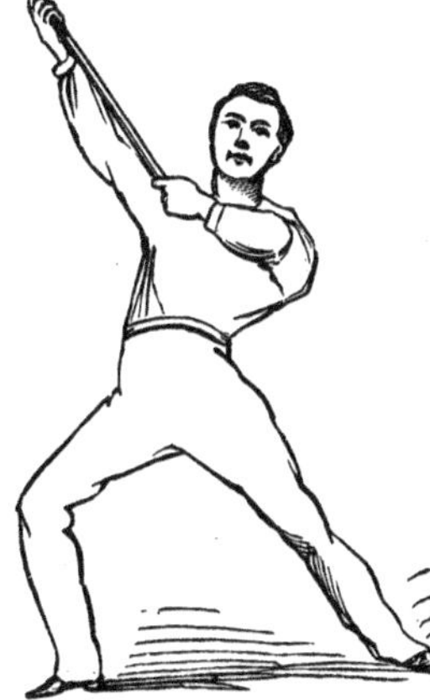

Figure 11.

No. 19. Same as the last, except when the right foot charges diagonally forward, the wand is made to point diagonally backwards over the left shoulder, and vice versa.

No. 20. Same as the last, except when the right foot charges diagonally forward, the wand is made to point diagonally backward, over the right shoulder, and when the left foot charges diagonally forward, the wand is made to point diagonally backward, over the left shoulder.

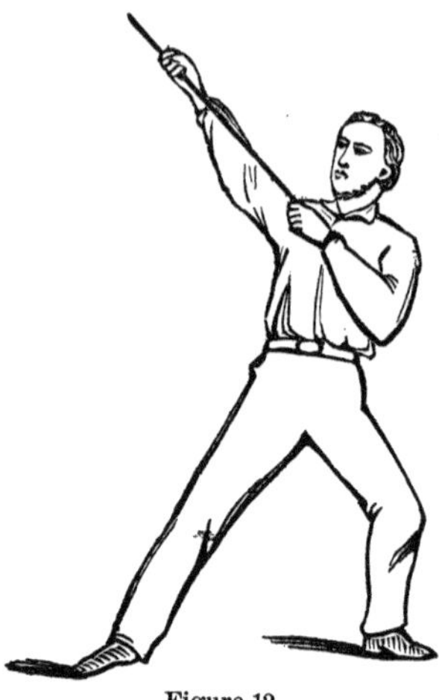

Figure 12.

No. 21. Same as the last, except the feet charge diagonally backward. As the left foot charges, thus, the wand is made to point diagonally forward, on the right side, and vice versa. (*Fig.* 12.)

No. 22. Same as the last, except when the left foot charges diagonally backward, the wand is made to point diagonally forward on the left side, and when the right foot charges diagonally backward, the wand points diagonally forward, on the right side.

No. 23. Same as the last, except when the left foot charges diagonally backward, the wand points diagonally backward, on the same side. And when the right foot charges diagonally backward, the wand points diagonally backward, on the same side.

No. 24. Same as the last, except when the left foot charges diagonally backward, on its own side, the wand points diagonally backward, on the right side, and vice versa.

It must not be forgotten that in all these compound exercises, involving the action of the arms and legs, the wand is always held at an angle of 45 degrees above the horizontal; and that in every case in passing from one charge to another, the wand is brought to the position represented in *Fig*. 8. Without this it would be impossible to keep time to the music. Let the steps be as long as possible.

No. 25. Wand horizontal over the head, as seen in *Fig*. 3. As in almost all the wand exercises, be careful not to bend the elbows. Turn the wand round so that the right hand comes exactly in front, and the left hand exactly behind. Bring the left in front and the right behind, so change twenty times.

No. 26. Hold the wand horizontal over the head, with the right hand in front and the left one behind. Make, by the side of the body, the motion seen in paddling a canoe. Each time carry the wand so far back that it shall be perpendicular. Do this ten times on the right side; then ten times on the left; then alternately ten times. Each time, as the wand is brought over the head it must be made horizontal, with one hand exactly in front, and the other behind, and as it is brought behind the body, it must be made perpendicular.

No. 27. Charge diagonally forward with the right foot; wand in the same direction. Left foot diagonally forward; wand the same. Left foot diagonally backward; wand the same. Right foot diagonally backward; wand the same. Having thus gone all around, begin again with the

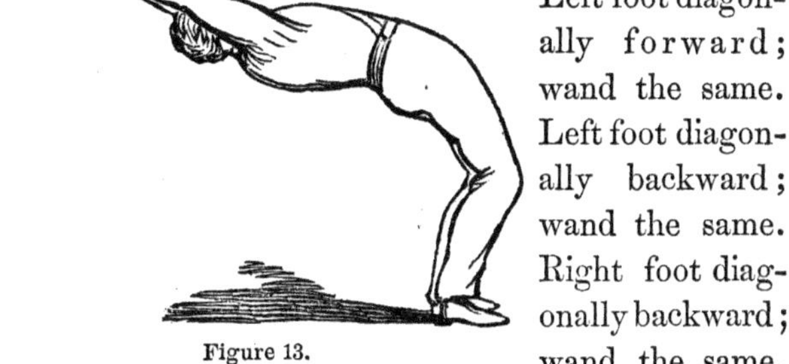

Figure 13.

left foot and go round the other way in like manner.

No. 28. With both hands take hold at the end of the wand. Hold it horizontal in front. Carry it directly backward without bending the arms, as seen in *Fig* 13. (I see the Artist has tipped the figure so far that the centre of gravity is lost.)

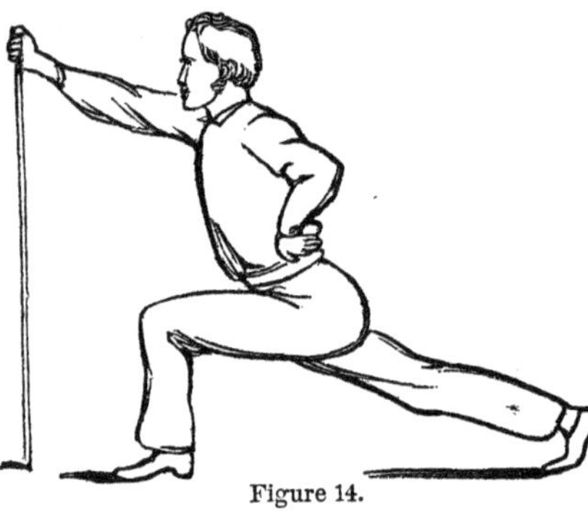

Figure 14.

No. 29. Heels together. Wand directly in front, resting on the floor, and perpendicular. Arm straight. Step the right foot forward to the wand, and back to the other foot, five times. Left foot the same.

No. 30. Step the right foot backward as far as you can reach, (*Fig*. 14.) and bring it back to the other foot, ten times. Same with the left foot.

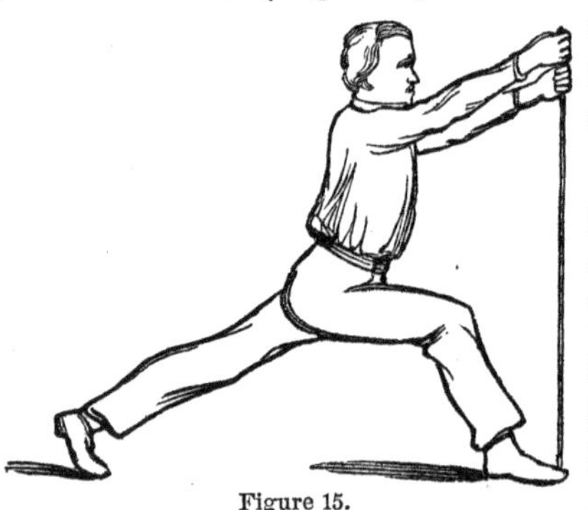

Figure 15.

No. 31. Carry the right foot forward to the wand. Returning, do not stop by the other foot, but carry it backward as far as you can reach. Now forward to the wand again. Make this long sweep ten times. Left foot the same.

No. 32. Seizing the upper end of the wand with both hands, as seen in *Fig*. 15, carry the right foot forward to the wand, and the left foot back as far as you can reach. Change them at a single jump, and so continue ten times.

No. 33. Hold the wand in the position seen in *Fig*. 9, on the right side, with the right hand at the lower end, and the left hand at the upper. Change it to the left side, with the left hand at the lower end, and the right hand at the upper; so change from side to side, ten times.

No. 34. Begin the same as in the last, except the wand is held on the back of the right shoulder instead of the front. Carry it now to the back of the left, and so alternate ten times.

No. 35. Beginning at the front of the right shoulder, as in No. 32, carry it to the front of the left shoulder. Then to the back of the left shoulder, and now to the back of the right shoulder. Go thus around the body five times.

No. 36. Begin at the front of the left shoulder, and go around the body the other way five times.

No. 37. Hold the wand on the front of the right shoulder. Carry it to the back of the left shoulder. Back again to the front of the right shoulder. Repeat ten times.

No. 38. Begin at the front of the left shoulder, and alternate with the back of the right shoulder.

No. 39. Again putting the wand in front, on the floor, perpendicular, with the right hand seizing the upper extremity, and the arm straight, step the right foot forward to the wand. Bring it back to the other foot. Now step sideways to the right as far as you can reach. Bring it back to the other foot again; now step backward as far as you can reach. Bring it back to the other foot. Still using the right foot, step sideways to the left as far as you can reach, passing it by the left leg behind, (*Fig.* 16.) now back to the other foot again. Pass it to the left again, in front of the left leg, (*Fig.* 17.) and bring it back to the other foot. Continue this round five times.

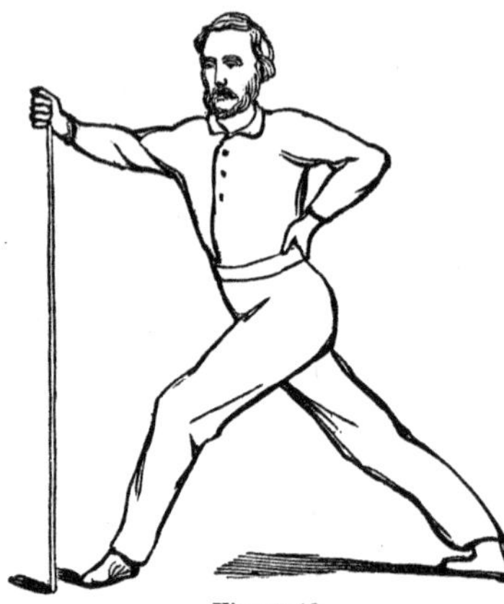

Figure 16.

No. 40. Same with the left arm and leg five times. In all this the wand must not loose its perpendicularity.

No. 41. Stand upright, with the heels together, seize the wand at its middle, with the right hand, and hold the arm horizontal in front—wand perpendicular. Keeping the arm in the horizontal place, whirl it round the body, making a complete circle, but do not stir the feet. Same with the left hand, ten times.

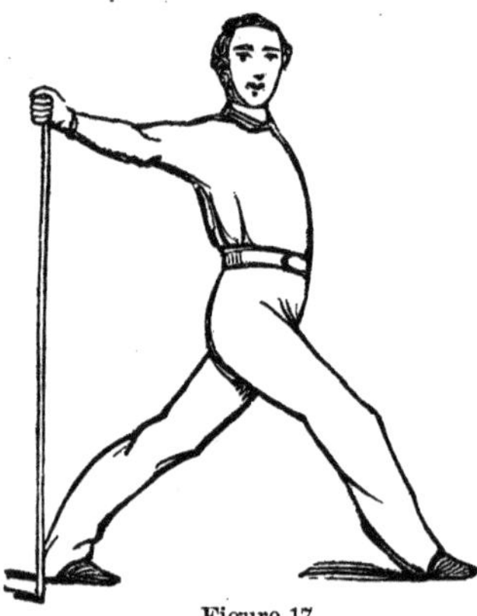

Figure 17.

No. 42. Grasp the middle of the wand with both hands, and whirl as in the last, as far as you can, ten times.

No. 43. Same as the last, except the wand is held horizontal, instead of perpendicular.

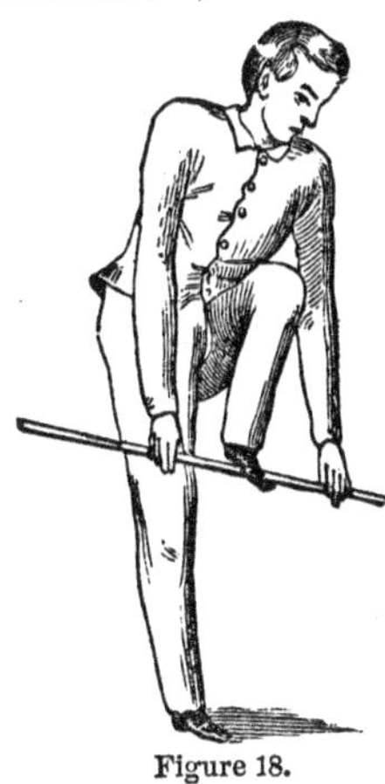
Figure 18.

No. 44. Seizing the wand as seen in *Fig.* 18, step backward and forward over it with the right and left foot, ten times.

No. 45. Stand upright, heels together, grasp the wand at the extreme ends and hold it behind the body, keeping the arms straight. The right hand high up, and the left hand low down. Now swing the left hand high up, and the right low down, and so continue to change the relative positions of the ends of the wand, without bending the elbows, ten times.

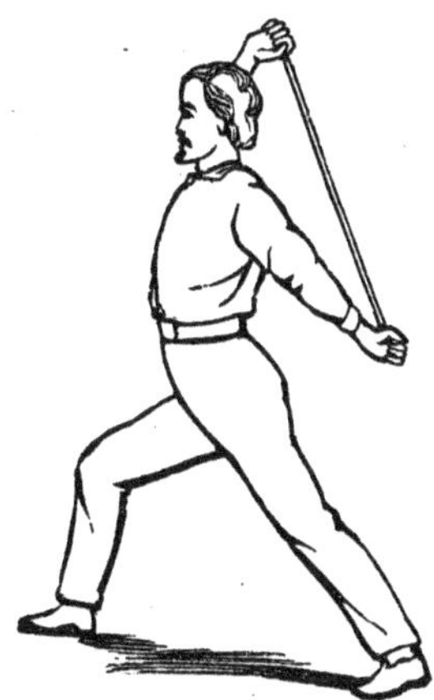
Figure 19.

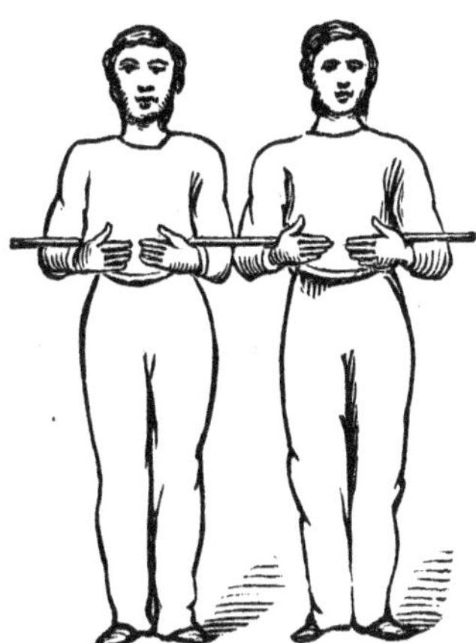
Figure 20.

No. 46. Charge the right foot diagonally forward, as seen in *Fig.* 19, five times. Now the left foot with the left hand raised high, five times. Alternate five times.

No. 47. Same as the last, except that when charging with the right foot, you raise the left hand high, and vice versa.

The wand exercises from this point are performed in couples, and while marching.

No. 48. Marching as represented in *Fig.* 20, leap sideways as far as possible, first one foot, and then the other, without loosing your relation to each other.

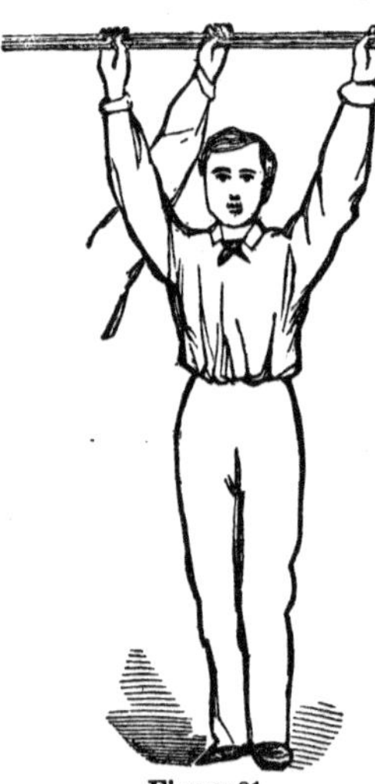
Figure 21.

No. 49. Putting the two wands together, and holding them as represented in *Fig.* 21, leap sideways as before, being sure to keep the shoulders back, and so leaping together, that the two will move as one person. Be sure to keep the arms quite perpendicular over the shoulders.

No. 50. One person walking directly behind the other, take hold of the extreme ends of the wands, and then allow the hands to rest on the shoulders. Marching in this way, at the word of command, "Up," raise the wands as high as you can, and as the right foot goes forward, thrust the right hand as far forward as possible, the left one at the same time being pushed as far back as possible, (*Fig.* 22.) and as the left foot comes forward reverse the hands.

No. 51. Same as the last, except the right hand

goes forward with the left foot, and the left hand with the right foot. In all these you must not bend the elbows, except when you are told to bend them.

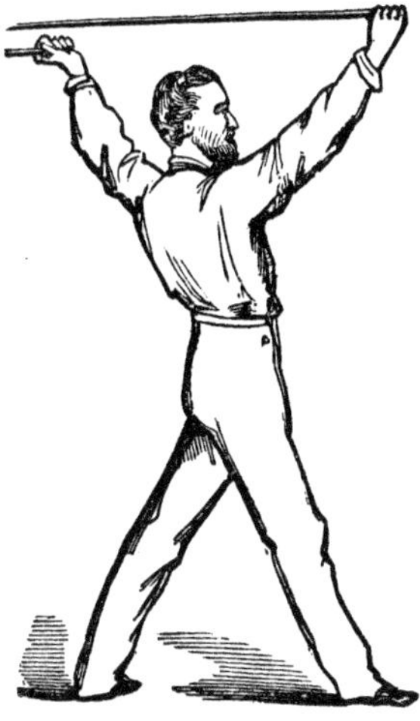

Figure 22.

No. 52. Still keeping your arms perpendicular, carry both of your hands forward as far as you can reach, with your right foot, and as you step your left foot forward, carry both hands as far back as you can reach, and thus continue for ten steps.

No. 53. Same as the last, except that the hands go forward with the left foot, and backward when the right foot goes forward.

No. 54. Bring the hands to the shoulders, and as the right foot steps forward, raise the right hands as high as you can reach. When the left foot goes forward raise the left hands, and bring down the right hands, and so continue to alternate ten times.

No. 55. Same as the last, except the right hands go up as the left feet go forward, and the left hands with the right feet.

No. 56. The two hands go up simultaneously with the stepping forward of the right feet, and come down as the left feet go forward.

No. 57. Same as the last, except the hands go up as the left feet go forward, and down as the right feet go forward. Be sure in the last four exercises that the arms go up and down quite vertically.

No. 58. Put the two wands together and take hold of them with one hand, as represented in *Fig.* 23, and marching side by side, leap sideways right and left, keeping the wand as high as you can reach.

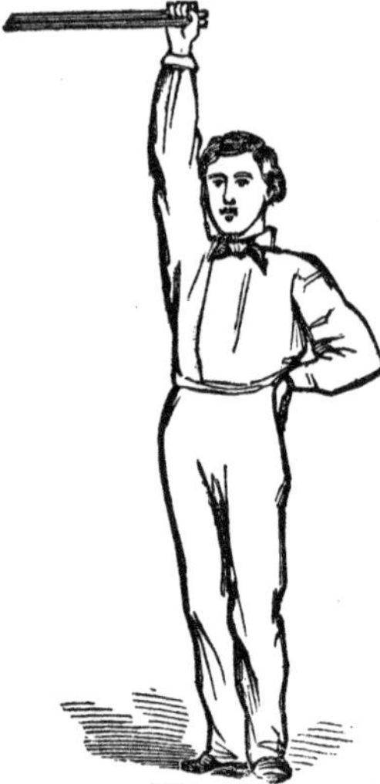
Figure 23.

No. 59. Partners change sides and repeat the same.

No. 60. Carrying the wands as in *Fig.* 23, as you step forward with the right foot, bring the wand down so as to strike your right leg with the hand, and then as your left foot goes forward, carry the wand back to its vertical position, and so continue ten times.

No. 61. Change sides with your partner, and do the same again, only bringing your wand down as the left foot goes forward, and raising it as the right foot goes forward.

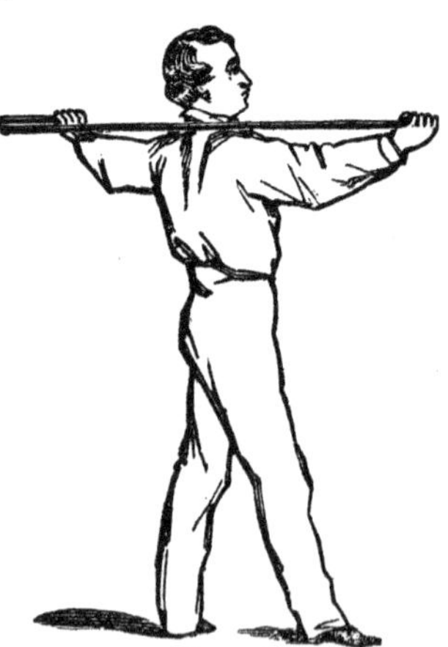
Figure 24.

No. 62. Cross the hands on the two wands placed side by side, but instead of holding them over the head, as in *Fig.* 21, let them hang down in front, and carrying them thus, leap from side to side.

No. 63. Walking one in front of the other, and extending the arms horizontally, *being careful not to bend the elbows*, carry the right forward as far as possible with the right foot, as represented in *Fig*. 24, and simultaneously with this, carry the left foot backward, as far as possible. When the left foot comes forward, let the left hand come forward too, and thus alternate.

No. 64. Same as the last, except that the right hand comes forward with the left foot, and vice versa.

No. 65. The same simultaneously with the right foot, and with the left foot.

Be careful in the performance of the last four, that you keep the arms exactly horizontal from first to last.

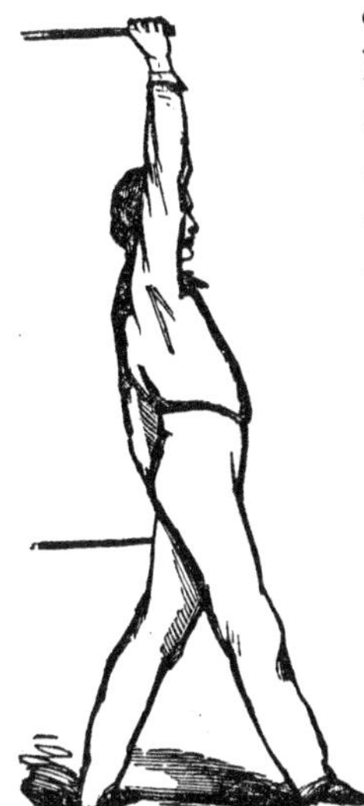
Figure 25.

No. 66. Walking, one in front of the other, with the wands hanging in the hands on either side, carry one up as high as you can reach, as in *Fig*. 25, and then as the other foot goes forward, carry up the other while the first is brought down.

No. 67. Same as last, except the right arms go up as the left foot goes forward, and vice versa.

No. 68. Simultaneously up with the right foot forward ten times, and the same with the left foot.

It is perhaps unnecessary to repeat that every motion with the wands is to be done to music. In making the changes from one exercise to another, this rule must not be forgotten.

It must not be forgotten that the feet, in every exercise, are to be kept at a right angle with each other.

It is hardly necessary to say that teachers may add to this series at pleasure. It is not difficult to extemporise a few exercises which are exactly adapted to some unusual circumstance, as for example a crowded room, or some peculiar position of the seats.

I have the wands made hollow sometimes, and loaded with a small mass of iron, or a pound or two of shot, which, moving from end to end, serves with a slight noise to mark the time, and add to the force of the exercises.

The shorter the wand the more difficult the exercise; so when a pupil has made some advance and feels himself competent to severer labor, direct him to seize the wand at a little distance from the end. By drawing in the hands a few inches at either end, he will add greatly to the difficulty of the feats.

If once a month the wands be well rubbed with sand paper, they will be kept smooth and neat.

DUMB BELL EXERCISES.

For more than two thousand years the dumb bell has been in use as a means of physical culture. It was highly prized by the Greeks. Many advantages are justly claimed in its behalf. If used in private, it occupies little space either at rest or in action. For the same reason it is excellent in the training of large classes. Although not to be compared with the New Gymnastic Ring, the Dumb Bell deserves its great popularity.

Among the Greeks it had a peculiar shape, and in this respect has undergone many changes, of which something will be said hereafter. Its present shape is well known. A practical suggestion upon this point may not be amiss. The handle should be at least half an inch longer than the width of the hand, of such size as can be easily grasped, with a slight swell in the middle. The manufacturer must not forget there is a wide difference between the hand of a little girl and that of a large man.

Heretofore dumb bells have been made of metals. The weight in this country has usually been considerable. The general policy at present is to employ those as heavy as the health seeker can put up. This is wrong. In the great German Gymnastic Institutes dumb bells were formerly employed weighing from fifty to one hundred pounds, but now, SCHREBER and other distinguished authors, condemn such weights and advocate those weighing from two to five pounds. I think those weighing two pounds are heavy enough for any man, and as it is important that they be of considerable size, I introduced some years ago, those made of wood. Every year my faith grows stronger in their superiority.

In my early experience as a teacher of Gymnastics I advocated heavy dumb bells, prescribing for those who could put up one hundred pounds, a bell of that weight. As my success had always been with heavy weights, pride led me to continue their use, long after I doubted the wisdom of such a course. For some years I have employed only those made of wood.

I know it will be said that dumb bells of two pounds weight will do for women and children, but can not answer the requirements of strong men.

The weight of the dumb bell turns entirely on the manner in which it is used. If only lifted over the head, one or two pounds would be absurdly light; but if used as we employ them, then one weighing ten pounds is beyond the strength of the strongest. No man can enter one of my classes of little girls even, and go through the exercises with bells weighing ten pounds each.

We had a good opportunity to laugh at a class of young men last year, who, upon entering the gymnasium organized an insurrection against the wooden dumb bells, and through a committee asked me to procure iron ones; I ordered a quantity weighing three pounds each; they used them part of one evening, and when asked the following evening, which they would have, replied, "the wooden ones will do."

A just statement of the issue is this: if you only lift the dumb bell from the floor, put it up, and then put it down again, of course it should be heavy, or there is no exercise; but if you would use it in a great variety of ways, assuming a hundred graceful attitudes, and bringing the muscles into use in every direction, requiring skill and followed by a harmonious development, the bell must be light.

There need be no controversy between the light weight and the heavy weight party on this point. We of the light weight party agree that if the bell is to be used as the heavy weight party uses it, it must be heavy; but if as we use it, then it must be light. If they of the heavy weight party think not, we only ask them to try it.

The only question which remains is that which lies between all heavy and light gymnastics, viz: whether strength or flexibility is to be preferred. Without entering upon a discussion of the physiological principles which underlie this subject, I will simply say that I prefer the latter. The Hanlon brothers and Heenan are, physiologically considered, greatly superior to heavy lifters.

But here I ought to say that no man can be flexible without a good degree of strength. It is not however, that kind of strength involved in great lifting. Heenan is a very strong man, can strike a blow twice as hard as Windship, but cannot lift seven hundred pounds nor put up an eighty-pound dumb bell. Wm. Hanlon, who is probably the finest gymnast, with the exception of Blondin, ever seen on this continent, cannot lift six hundred pounds. Such men have a great fear of lifting. They know almost by instinct that it spoils their muscles.

One of the finest gymnasts in the country told me

that in several attempts to lift five hundred pounds he failed, and that he should never try it again. This same gymnast owns a fine horse. Ask him to lend that horse to draw before a cart and he will refuse, because such labor would make the animal stiff, and unfit him for light, graceful movements before the carriage.

The same physiological law holds true of man; lifting great weights affects him as drawing heavy loads affects the horse. So far from man's body being an exception to this law, it bears with peculiar force upon him. Moving great weights through small spaces, produces a slow, inelastic, inflexible man. No matter how flexible a young man may be, let him join a circus company, and lift the cannon twice a day, for two or three years, and he will become as inflexible as a cart horse. No matter how elastic the colt is when first harnessed to the cart, he will soon become so inelastic that he is unfit to serve before the carriage.

Men, women and children should be strong, but it should be the strength of grace, flexibility, agility and endurance; it should not be the strength of a great lifter. I alluded to the gymnastics of the circus. Let all who are curious in regard to the point I am discussing, visit it. Permit me to call special attention to three features—to the man who lifts the cannon, to the india-rubber man, and to the general performer.

The lifter and the india-rubber man constitute the two mischievous extremes. It is impossible that in either there should be the highest physiological conditions; but in the persons of the Hanlon brothers, who are general performers, is found the model gymnast. They can neither lift great weights nor tie themselves into knots, but they occupy a point between these two extremes. They possess both strength and flexibility, and resemble fine, active, agile, vigorous carriage horses, which occupy a point between the slow cart horse and the long-legged, loose-jointed animal.

With heavy dumb bells the extent of motions is very slight, and of course the range and freedom of action will be correspondingly so. This is a point of great importance. The limbs, and indeed the entire body, should have the widest and freest range of motion. It is only thus that our performances in the business or pleasures of life become most effective. A complete, equable circulation of the blood is thereby most perfectly secured. And this, I may remark, is in one aspect the physiological purpose of all exercise. The race horse has a much more vigorous circulation than the cart horse. It is a fact not unfamiliar with horsemen, that when a horse is transferred from slow, heavy work to the carriage, the surface veins about the neck and legs begin at once to enlarge; when the change is made from the carriage to the cart, the reverse is the result.

And when we consider that the principal object of all physical training is an elastic, vigorous condition of the nervous system, the superiority of light gymnastics becomes still more obvious. The nervous system is the fundamental fact of our earthly life. All other parts of the organism exist and work for it. It controls all and is the seat of pain and pleasure.

The impressions upon the stomach, for example, resulting in a better or worse digestion, must be made through the nerves. This supreme control of the nervous system is forcibly illustrated in the change made by joyful or sad tidings.

The overdue ship is believed to have gone down with her valuable, uninsured cargo. Her owner paces the wharf, sallow and wan; appetite and digestion gone. She heaves in sight! She lies at the wharf! The happy man goes aboard, hears all is safe, and, taking the officers to a hotel, devours with them a dozen monstrous compounds, with the keenest appetite, and without a subsequent pang.

I am confident that the loyal people of this country have eaten and digested, since Roanoke and Donelson, as they had not before since Sumpter.

Could we have an unbroken succession of good news, we should all have good digestion without a gymnasium. But in a world of vexation and disappointment, we are driven to the necessity of muscle culture, and other hygienic expedients, to give the nervous system that support and vitality, which our fitful surroundings deny.

If we would make our muscle training contributive in the highest degree to the healthful elasticity of our nerves, the exercises must be such, as will bring into varied combinations and play all our muscles and nerves. Those exercises which require great accuracy, skill and dash, are just those which secure this happy and complete intermarriage of nerve and muscle. If any one doubts that boxing and small sword will do more to give elasticity and tone to the nervous system, than lifting kegs of nails, then I will give him over to the heavy lifters.

Another point I take the liberty to urge. Without *accuracy* in the performance of the feats, the interest must be transient. This principle is strikingly exemplified in military training. Those who have studied our infantry drill, have been struck with its simplicity, and have wondered that men could go through with its details every day for years, without disgust. If the drill master permit carelessness, then, authority alone can force the men through the evolutions; but if he enforce the greatest precision, they return to their task every morning, for twenty years, with fresh and increasing interest.

What precision, permit me to ask, is possible in "putting up" a heavy dumb-bell? But in the new dumb bell exercises, there is opportuniy and necessity for all the accuracy and skill which are found in the most elaborate military drills.

I have been a teacher of boxing and fencing, and I say with confidence, that in neither or both is there such a field for fine posturing, wide, graceful action, and studied accuracy, as is to be found in the new series of dumb bell exercises.

But, it is said, if you use bells weighing only two pounds, you must work an hour to reach the exercise which the heavy ones would furnish in five minutes. I need not inform those who have practiced the new series with the light bells, that this objection is made in ignorance. If you simply "put up" the light bell, it is true, but if you use it as herein described and illustrated, it is not true. On the contrary, in less than five minutes, legs, hips, back, arms, shoulders, neck, lungs and heart, will each and all make the most emphatic remonstrance against even a quarter of an hour's practice of such feats.

At this point it may be urged that those exercises which hasten the action of the thoracic viscera, to any considerable degree, are simply exhaustive. This is another blunder of the "big muscle" men. They seem to think you can determine every man's constitution and health, by the tape line; and that all exercises whose results are not determinable by measurement are worthless.

I need scarcely say, there are certain conditions of brain, muscle and of every other tissue, far more important than size; but what I desire to urge more particularly in this connection, is the importance, the great physiological advantages, of just those exercises in which the lungs and heart are brought into active play. These organs are no exceptions to the law that exercise is the principal condition of development.—Their vigorous training adds more to the stock of vitality, than that of other organs. A man may stand still and lift kegs of nails and heavy dumb bells until his shoulders and arms are Sampsonian, he will contribute far less to his health and longevity, than by a daily run of a mile or two.

Speaking in a general way, those exercises in which the lungs and heart are made to go at a vigorous pace, are to be ranked among the most useful. The "double-quick" of the soldier contributes more in five minutes to his digestion and endurance, than the ordinary drill in two hours.

I have said an elastic tone of the nervous system is the physiological purpose of all physical training. If one may be allowed such an analysis, I would add that we exercise our muscles to invigorate the thoracic and abdominal viscera. These in their turn support and invigorate the nervous system. All exercises which operate more directly upon these internal organs,—as for example, laughing, deep breathing and running, contribute most effectively to the stamina of the brain and nerves.

It is only this mania for monstrous arms and shoulders that could have misled the intelligent gymnast on this point.

But finally, it is said, you certainly cannot deny that rapid motions with great sweep, exhaust more than slow motions through limited spaces. A great lifter said to me the other day, "do you pretend to deny that a locomotive with a light train, flying at the rate of forty miles an hour, consumes more fuel than one with a heavy train, moving at the rate of five miles?" I did not attempt to deny it. "Well then," he added with an air of triumph, "what have you to say now about these great sweeping feats with your light dumb bells, as compared with the slow putting up of heavy ones?"

I replied by asking him another question. "Do you pretend to deny that when you drive your horse ten miles within an hour, before a light carriage, he is more exhausted than by drawing a load two miles an hour?" "That's my doctrine exactly," he said. Then I asked, "why don't you always drive two miles an hour?" "But my patients would all die," replied my friend. I did not say aloud what was passing in my mind—that the danger to his patients might be less than he imagined; but I suggested, that nearly every man as well as every horse, had duties in this life which involved the necessity of rapid and vigorous motions. That were this slow movement generally adopted, every phase of human life would be stripped of progress, success and glory.

As our artificial training is designed to fit us for the more successful performance of the business of life, I suggest that the training should be, in character, somewhat assimilated to those duties. If you would train a horse for the carriage, you would not prepare him by driving at a slow pace before a heavy load. If you did, the first fast drive would go hard with him.

Just so with a man. If he is to lift hogsheads of sugar, or kegs of nails, as a business, he may be trained by heavy lifting; but if his business requires the average velocity and free motions of human occupations, then upon the basis of his heavy, slow training, he will find himself in actual life, in the condition of the dray horse, who is pushed before the light carriage at a high speed.

Perhaps it is not improper to add, that to me, all this talk about expenditure of vitality is full of sophistry. Teachers and writers speak of our stock of vitality, as if it were a vault of gold, upon which you cannot draw without lessening the quantity. Whereas, it is rather like the mind or heart enlarging by action, gaining by expenditure.

When Daniel Boone was living alone in Kentucky, his intellectual exercises were doubtless of the quiet, slow, heavy character. Other white men joined him. Under the social stimulus, his thinking became more sprightly. Suppose that in time he had come to write vigorously, and to speak in the most eloquent, brilliant manner, does any one imagine that he would have lost in mental vigor and dash by the process? Would not the brain, which had only slow exercise in his isolated life, become bold, brilliant and dashing, by bold, brilliant and dashing efforts?

A farm boy has slow, heavy muscles. He has been accustomed to heavy exercises. He is transferred to the circus, and performs, after a few years training, a hundred beautiful, splendid feats! He at length reaches the matchless Zampillærstation of Wm. Hanlon. Does any one think that his body has lost power in this brilliant education?

Is it true that in either intellectual or physical training, bold, brilliant efforts, under proper conditions and limitations, exhaust the powers of life? On the contrary, is it not true that we find in vigorous, bold, dashing, brilliant efforts, the only source of vigorous, bold, dashing and brilliant powers?

In this discusion I have not considered the treatment of invalids. The principles presented are applicable to the training of children and adults of average vitality.

In a work upon which I am now engaged, devoted to the "Movement Cure," to be published early in 1863, I shall advocate, and for reasons which will appear in the work, an entirely different policy.

In the mean time I will rest upon the general statement, that all persons of both sexes, and of every age, who are possessed of average vitality, should, in the department of physical education, employ light apparatus, and execute a great variety of feats, which require skill, accuracy, courage, dash, presence of mind, quick eye and hand—in brief, which demand a vigorous and complete exercise of all the powers and faculties with which the Creator has endowed us.

While deformed and diseased persons should be treated in consonance with the philosophy of the *Swedish Movement Cure*, in which the movements are slow and limited.

It is but justice to the following series of exercises with dumb bells, as well as to myself, to state that not only are they, with two or three exceptions, my own invention, but the wisdom of the precise arrangement given, as well as the balance of exercise in all the muscles of the body and limbs, have been well proven by an extensive use for several years.

It must not be forgotten that in all the dumb bell exercises the pupil should, as a beginning position, stand with his heels together, the toes separated so as to make between the feet a right angle, and the arms hanging by the sides with the dumb bells horizontal, and parallel to each other.

Not only in all the exercises but in all the changes from one exercise to another, the pupil must keep time to the music. In the absence of other musical instruments a drum may be employed to mark the time; and even without this it may be kept by counting one, two; one, two; one, two.

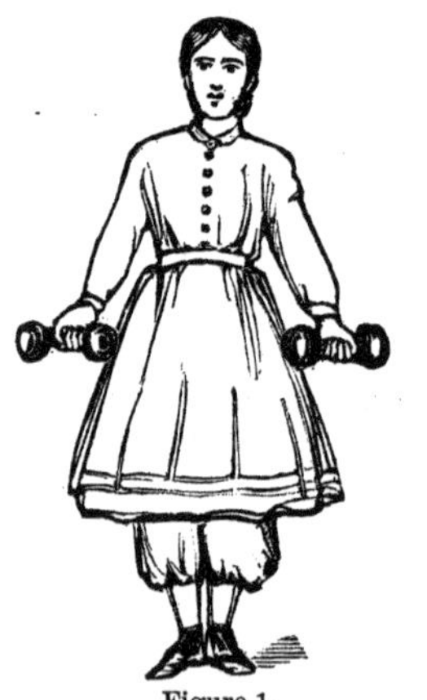
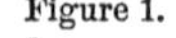

Figure 1.

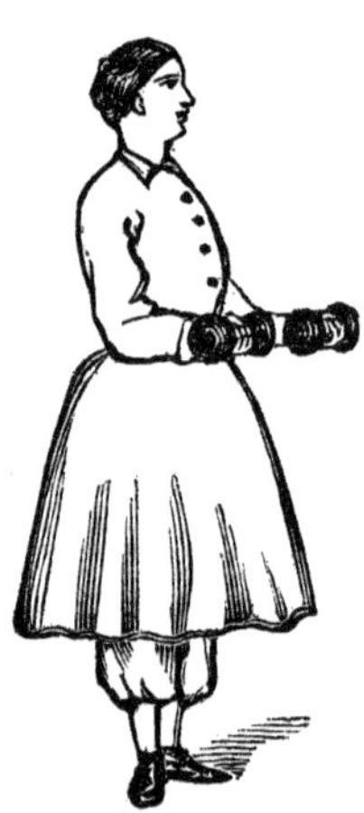

Figure 2.

It must be remembered that in no case should the pupil bend the legs at the knee, or his arms at the elbow, unless it is so directed. No rule in the dumb bell exercises is so important as this. If it be forgotten, exercises with dumb bells will loose more than half their value.

No. 1. The position is shown in *Fig*. 1. Thumbs outward. Bells *exactly horizontal*. Turn the thumb ends of the bells to the hips, and then back again to the position shown in the figure. *Repeat ten times*. Let the change be made with the greatest accuracy. When it is well done, no matter which end is at the hip, a straight rod run through one dumb bell, lengthwise, would at the same time run through the centre of the other.

In this and all subsequent dumb bell exercises, the pupil must be careful not to bend the elbows. When exceptions to this rule occur, they will be plainly indicated.

No. 2. Position seen in *Fig*. 2. Keep the elbows pressed against the sides, and twist the bells so the ends are exactly reversed. Be sure they are exactly in line with each other, and the forearms parallel. *Repeat ten times*.

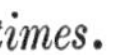

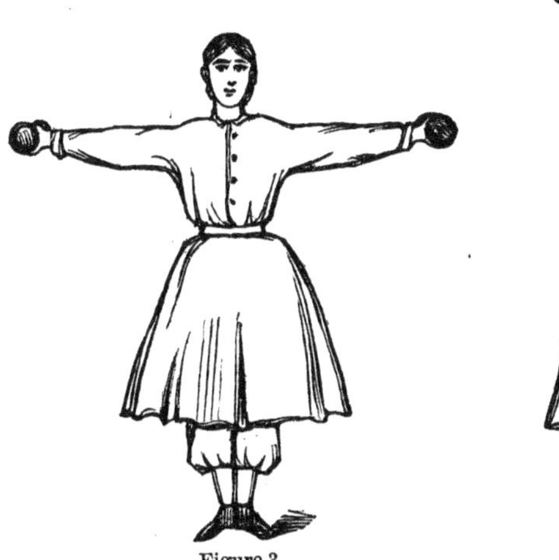

Figure 3.

Figure 4.

No. 3. In passing from No. 2 to No. 3, bring the bells to the chest, and on the next beat to the position in *Fig.* 3. The palms of the hands are upward. Bells exactly horizontal and parallel to each other. Turn the hands over, knuckles upward. Bells now exactly in the same position as before. *Repeat ten times.*

No. 4. In passing from No. 3 to No. 4, bring the bells to the chest, and on the next beat to the position in *Fig.* 4. The palms forward. Twist the bells so the knuckles are forward. *Repeat ten times.* Arms to be kept parallel from first to last.

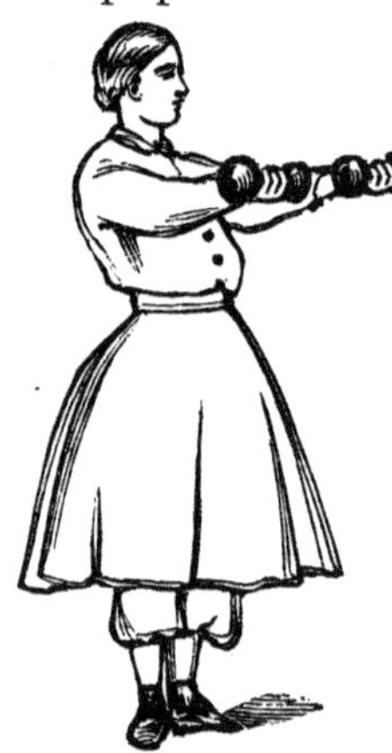
Figure 5.

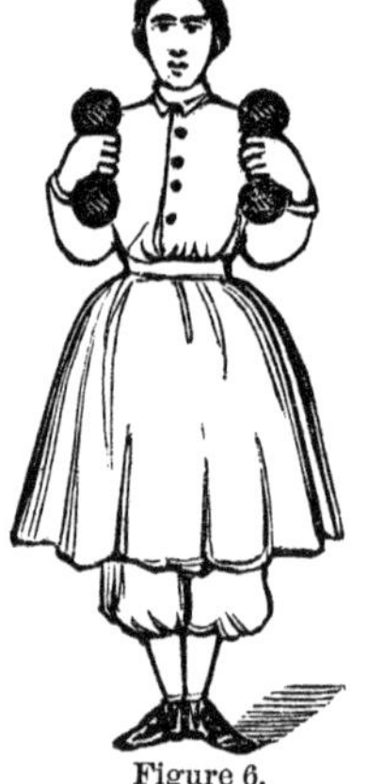
Figure 6.

No. 5. Position as in *Fig.* 5. In passing from No. 4 to No. 5, bring the bells to the chest. Twist the arms so that the bells are exactly reversed.

It will be seen in the figure, the palms are upward. When the bells are reversed, the knuckles are upward. Keep the arms parallel. *Repeat ten times.*

In passing from one exercise to another, I have spoken of bringing the bells to the chest. They should strike the chest exactly at the point shown in *Fig.* 6.

No. 6. Thrust the two bells down by the side of the legs. Bring to the chest, and thrust them sideways. Bring to the chest and thrust them upward. Bring to the chest and thrust them forward.

Repeat these four thrusts five times.

When the down thrust is made, the pupil must be careful that at the lowest point the bells are precisely horizontal, and parallel to each other. When the side thrust is made the arms must be horizontal, the bells perpendicular and parallel to each other. When the upward thrust is made the arms must be accurately perpendicular, bells parallel and horizontal.

When the forward thrust is executed the arms must be exactly horizontal, and the bells perpendicular and parallel.

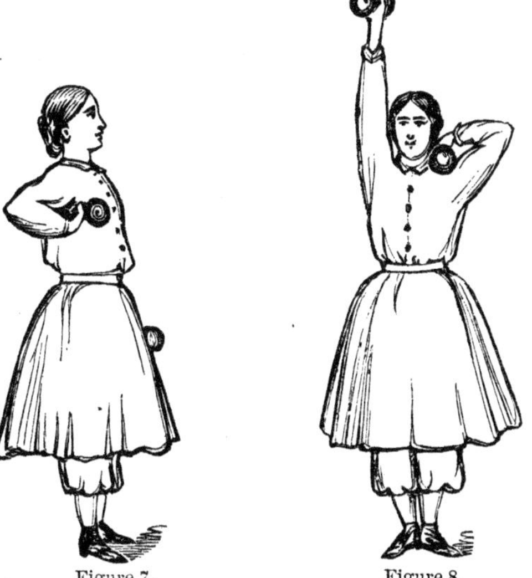

Figure 7. Figure 8.

No. 7. Raise the right hand bell from the side of

the leg into the arm-pit, five times. *(Fig. 7.)* Left, five times. Alternately and simultaneously, five times.

Be sure that each time when the bells come into the arm-pits they are exactly horizontal.

No. 8. Passing from No. 7, to No. 8, bring the bells to the chest; on the next beat, to the top of the shoulders; on the next beat carry up the right, reaching accurately the position seen in *Fig.* 8. *Repeat five times.* Left, the same. Alternately and simultaneously, each *five times.*

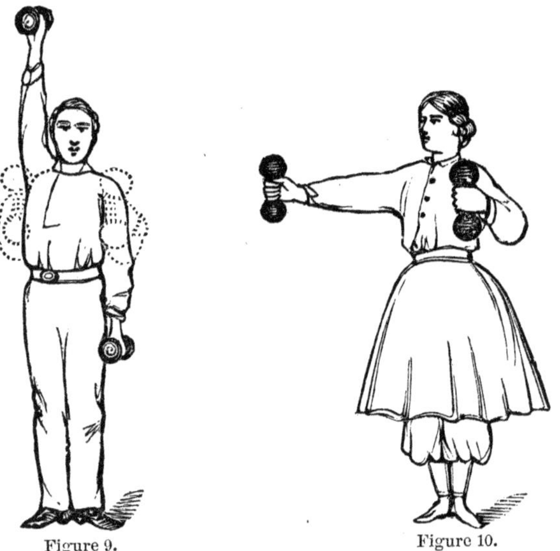

Figure 9. Figure 10.

No. 9. Passing from No. 8 to No 9, bring the bells to the chest, (the dotted lines in *Fig.* 9 show it) then down by the sides, in all, as usual, keeping good time to the music. Now carry the right bell to the chest, then up, reaching the position shown in *Fig.* 9. Return to the hip, marking one beat on the chest in going down. *Repeat ten times.* Left, the same. Alternately and simultaneously *ten times.*

No. 10. Bring the bells to the chest. Strike out the right one in front, arm precisely horizontal, bell perpendicular. (*Fig.* 10.) *Repeat twenty times.* Left, the same. Alternately and simultaneously, *twenty times.*

As usual, keep the chest well forward, and the shoulders drawn far back.

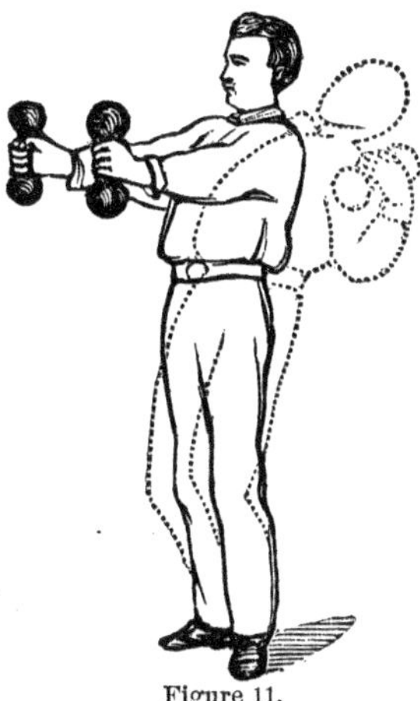
Figure 11.

No. 11. Holding the bells in the position seen in *Fig.* 11, bring them with *great force* into the position seen in the dotted line, forty times. In beginning this elbow thrust backward, it is well to first raise the bells a foot, that they may be brought back with more force, and more directly into the position seen in the dotted lines. But in carrying them forward again, it should be first into the position seen in the figure.

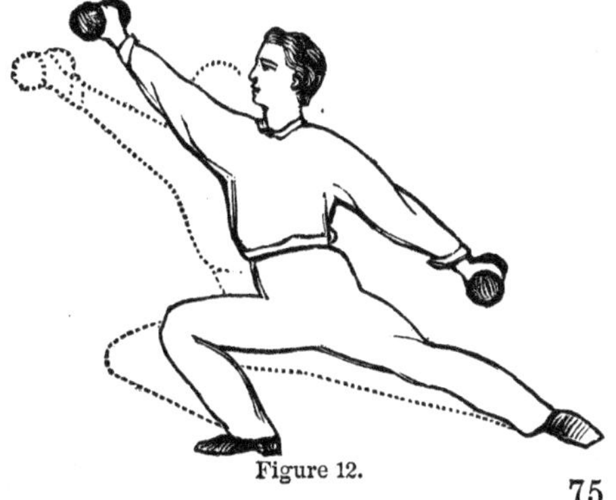
Figure 12.

No. 12. Stamp the left foot, then the right, then charge out into the position seen in *Fig.* 12. Making sure that the leg left behind, *in this and all subsequent charges*, is kept entirely straight, while the one forward is placed as shown in the figure. Holding the arms as illustrated, foıce the entire person into the position of the dotted lines, five times. *There should be no motion in the shoulder joints. The chest is pushed far forward, and the shoulders drawn well back.* These directions are applicable to all charging exercises, in which a different course is not plainly indicated.

It will be observed that the charge in No. 12 is exactly sideways.

Rise to the perpendicular again, stamp the right foot, then the left, and lastly charge out on the left side, and repeat the performance of the right side, *five times.*

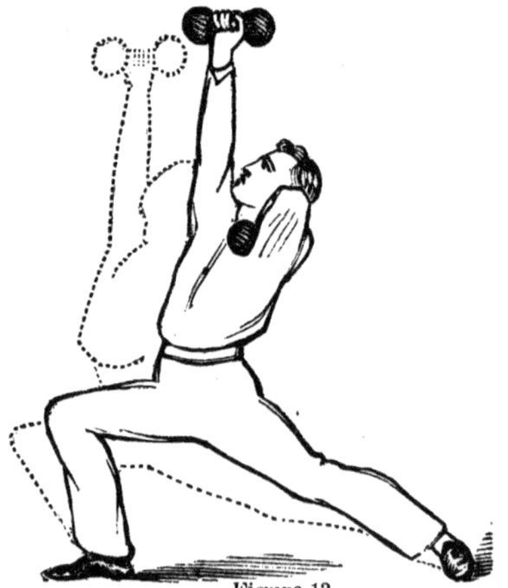

Figure 13.

No. 13. Rise to the perpendicular, stamp with the left foot, then with the right, then charge out as shown in *Fig.* 13. Under the directions given in No. 12, sink five times.

Same on the left side, of course with the intermedi-ate stamping.

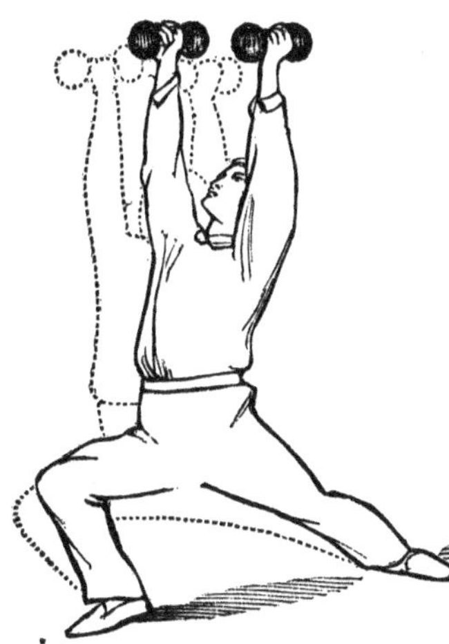

Figure 14.

No. 14. After the regular stamping, the pupil should charge in the manner illustrated in *Fig.* 14.

Sink five times.

Same on the left side.

In this, as in *Figs.* 12 and 13, the charging is exactly sideways.

No. 15. Stand upright, hands by the side. Raise the right hand as shown in *Fig.* 15, five times. Left the same. Alternately and simultaneously, five times.

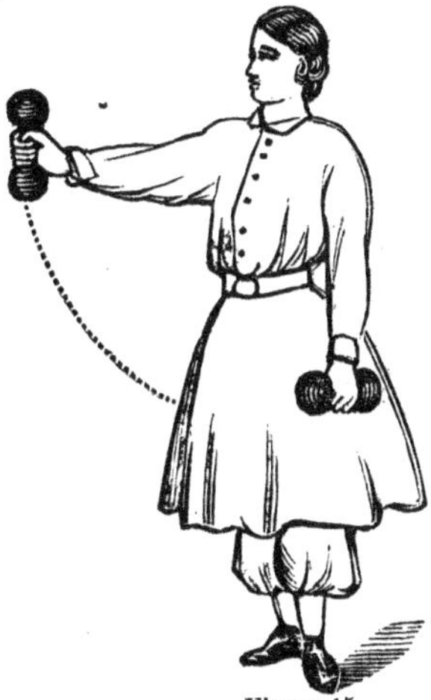

Figure 15.

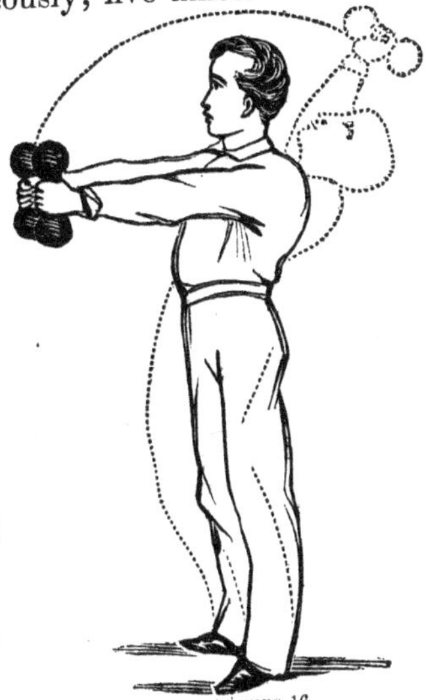

Figure 16.

In this the arm is carried up with a quick, strong effort, and arrested at the horizontal line, precisely as if it had struck a rock. When it is brought back to the side again, it is with the same force and sudden arrest. This and the next one are among the most severe of the dumb bell exercises.

No. 16. Assuming the position seen in *Fig.* 16, force back the right arm as seen in the dotted line, five times. Left the same. Alternately and simultaneously, five times.

The arm must not be bent at the elbow.

The directions given in No. 15, in regard to force and sudden arrest, are applicable to this exercise.

No. 17. Beginning as in No. 15, with the arms hanging, combine the two exercises, Nos. 15 and 16, in one sweep, reaching the position of the dotted line in *Fig.* 16. Repeat five times. Left hand the same. Alternately and simultaneously, five times.

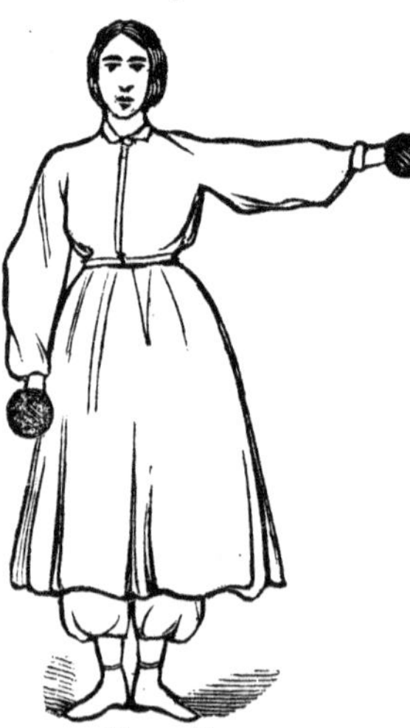
Figure 17.

No. 18. Stand upright, arms hanging. Raise the right arm to the horizontal, at the side, with the palm up. Repeat five times. Left, the same. Alternately and simultaneously, five times.—The position of one of the arms is seen in *Fig.* 17.

No. 19. Having the arms extended at the sides as shown in *Fig.* 18, raise the right arm to the position seen in the dotted line, five times.

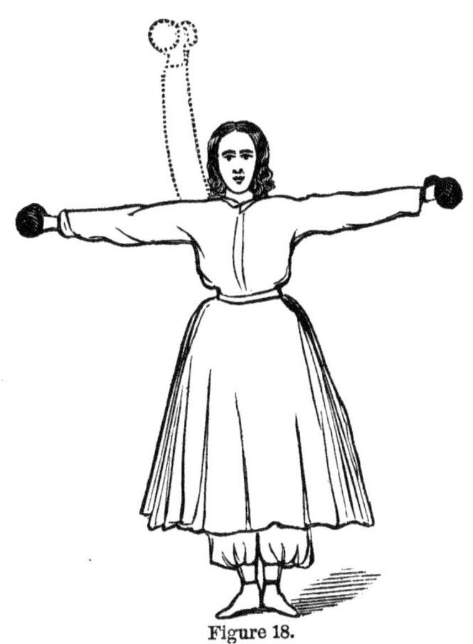

Figure 18.

Left, the same. Alternately and simultaneously, five times.

In raising the dumb bells over the head, be careful that they are in such a position that when the two are up together, they are exactly horizontal and parallel to each other.

No. 20. Beginning as in No. 18, arms hanging, combine Nos. 17 and 18, in one sweep, each arm five times. Alternately and simultaneously, the same.

No. 21. Standing upright, arms hanging, charge into the position shown in *Fig*. 19; remaining thus, thrust the arms in front in a horizontal line five times, alternately and simultaneously. Rising to the perpendicular, stamp with the right foot, then the left, then charge out with the left foot, and repeat the exercises with the arms.

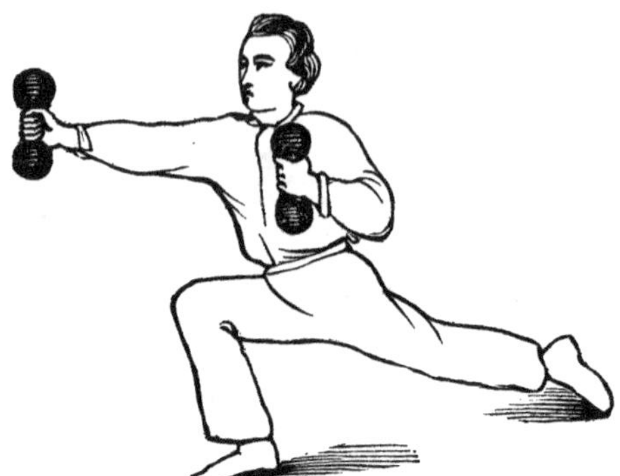

Figure 19.

It will be seen by the figure, that the leg behind is kept entirely straight and rests on the toe. The special point in this exercise is to reach the dumb bell as far forward as possible.

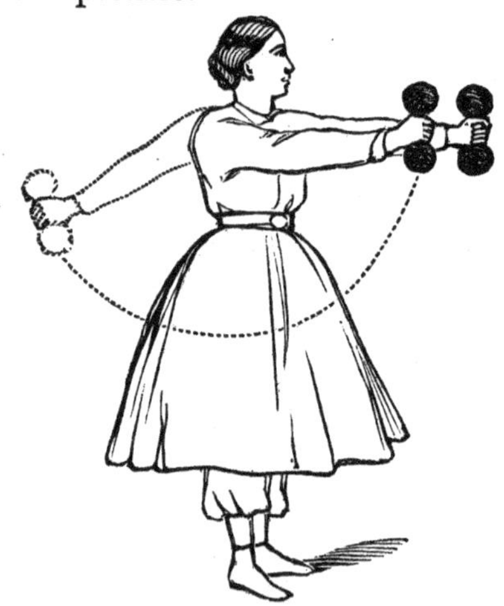

Figure 20.

No. 22. Standing as represented in *Fig.* 20, force the right arm into the position shown in the dotted line, five times. Left the same. Alternately and simultaneously five times.

In this exercise keep the body as erect as possible.

No. 23. Having the arms perpendicular over the head, perform the same exercise as in the last number, with right hand, left hand, then alternately and simultaneously.

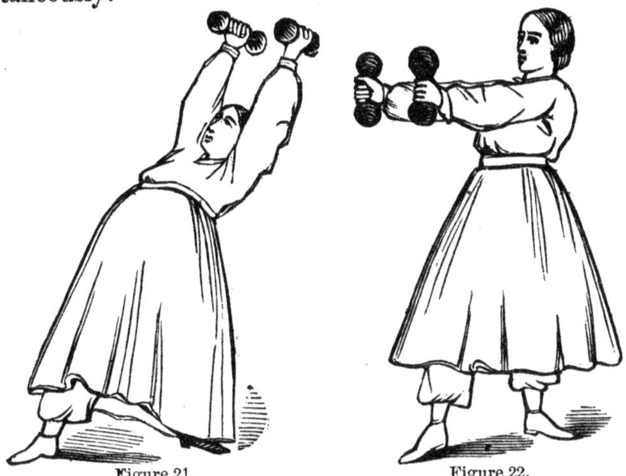

Figure 21. Figure 22.

No. 24. Placing the feet in the position of *Fig.* 21, raise the arms with great force from the hanging position to that seen in *Fig.* 21. On the next beat bring the arms to the position seen in *Fig.* 22; on the next

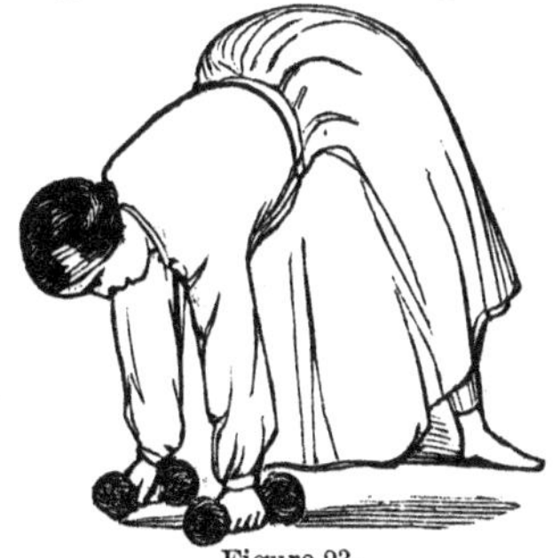

Figure 23.

to that seen in *Fig.* 23; on the next beat sweep back

to the position seen in *Fig.* 22; then to the position seen in *Fig.* 21. *Repeat five times.* Stamp right and left, then step out with the left foot, then swing the arms over the head, performing the same exercise on the left side.

In this exercise, neither arms nor legs should be bent.

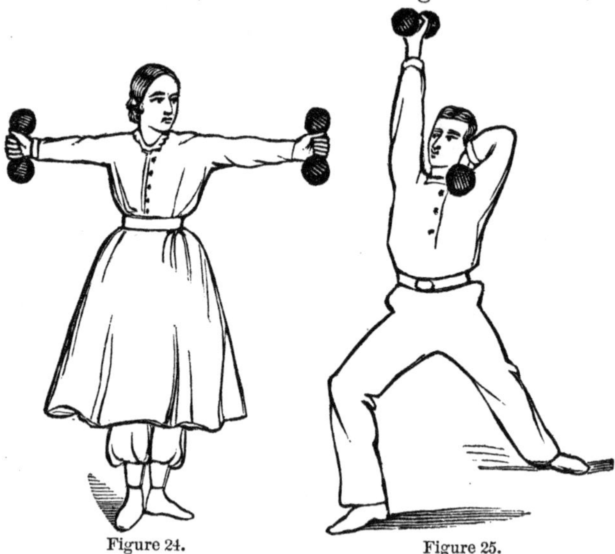

Figure 24. Figure 25.

No. 25. Stand erect, arms horizontal in front and parallel to each other. Carry the right hand backward in the horizontal plane (*Fig.* 24.) as far as possible; return it. Repeat ten times. Left the same; alternately and simultancously, ten times.

No. 26. Standing erect, arms hanging, stamp with the left foot; then with the right; then charge into the position seen in *Fig.* 25, and thrust the arms in a direct line upward, alternately and simultaneously ten times. Assuming the erect position drop the arms by the side, stamp the right foot, then the left, and charge out on the left side; repeat the exercise with the arms.

In this exercise, it will be seen, the leg behind is straight, that charged forward, considerably bent.

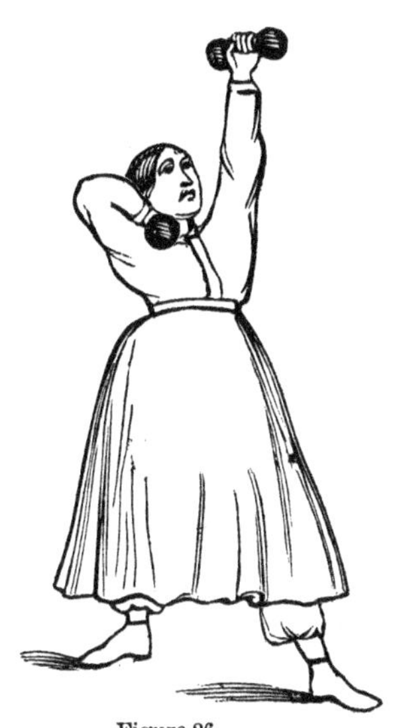
Figure 26.

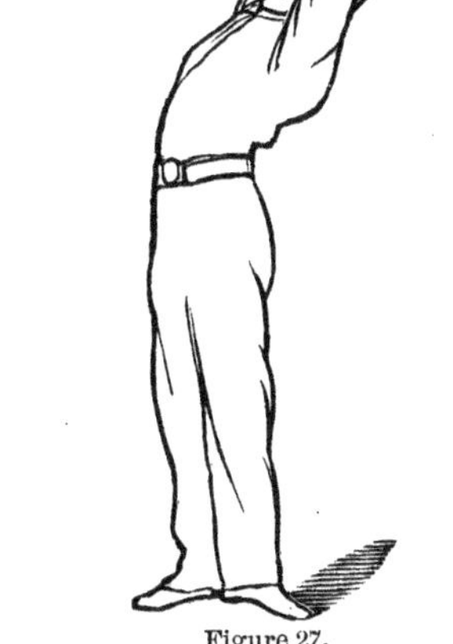
Figure 27.

No. 27. As in nearly all other exercises, begin with the heels together, body erect, chest forward, shoulders back, arms hanging, dumb bells horizontal and parallel to each other. Step diagonally backward with the right foot, as seen in *Fig.* 26, and repeat the exercises in No. 26. Same with the left foot.

In this exercise the forward leg is kept straight, that behind is bent as much as possible.

No. 28. Bells on the chest. Carry the right arm out at the side, thrusting it as far back as possible; suddenly bring it back to the chest in a circle as if grasping a large body standing in front. Repeat five times. Left hand, same. Alternately and simultaneously, same.

In this exercise the arms should be kept in the horizontal plane, and should in the performance of the exercise enclose as large an armful of the imaginary objects as possible.

No. 29. Standing erect, arms hanging at the side, suddenly turning the body to one side as far as you can twist it without moving the feet, carry the arms to the position seen in *Fig.* 27. Bring them back to the sides, while at the same time you bring the body to the first position. Swing the arms up on the other side, and so continue, alternating twenty times.

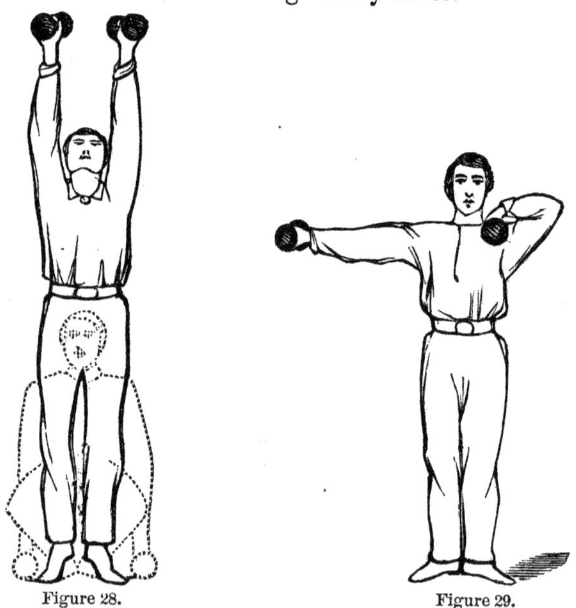

Figure 28. Figure 29.

No. 30. Standing erect, arms hanging, bring the bells to the chest, then to the floor, as shown in the dotted line in *Fig.* 28; then rising, bring the dumb bells again to the chest, and on the next beat thrust them as far upward as possible, rising on the toes; then back to the chest. Repeat twenty times.

No. 31. Standing erect, dumb bells on the shoulders, (not on the chest) thrust the right arm out at the side as seen in *Fig*. 29, ten times. Left the same. Alternately and simultaneously the same.

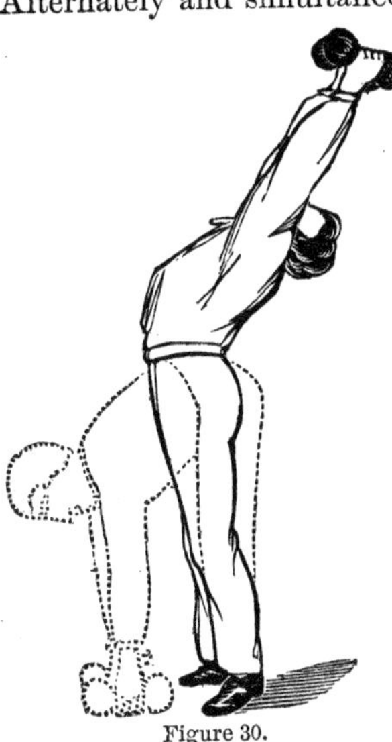
Figure 30.

No. 32. Standing erect, arms hanging, carry the arms to the horizontal in front; then to the position over the head seen in *Fig*. 30; now down to the horizontal again, and then to the floor as seen in the dotted line. Repeat ten times.

In this exercise there must be no bending at the knees or elbows.

No. 33. Standing erect, arms hanging, charge out with the right foot, and sweep the left arm as shown in *Fig*. 31; on the next beat return to the first position. Repeat five times. Same on the left side. Alternately, five times.

No. 34. Standing erect, arms hanging, without moving the body, carry the right foot out sideways, lifting it from the floor, and bringing it back to the other foot, without bending the knee, five times; then charge into the position seen in *Fig*. 32, and return to the first position, five times. Same on the left side. Alternately, five times.

The arm which is brought over the head, must be

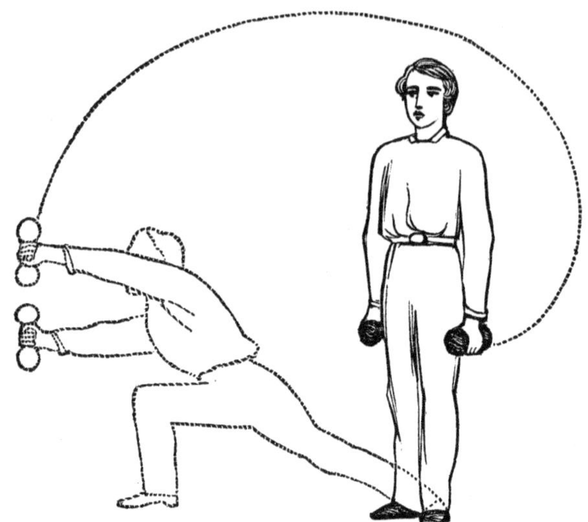

Figure 31.

carried in a direct line from the side, to the position over the head, and not brought toward the front of the body, in its passage up or down.

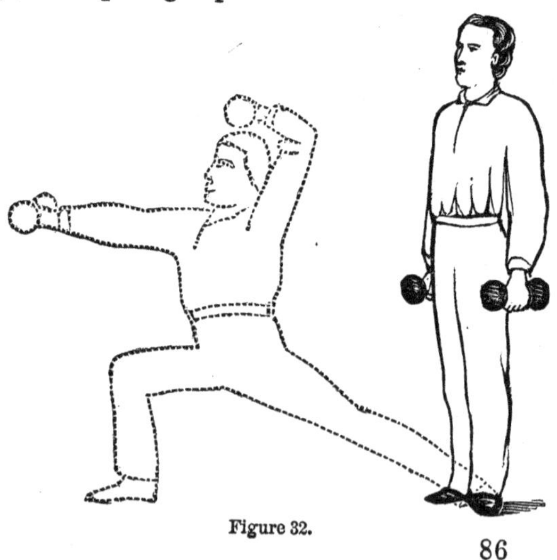

Figure 32.

CLUB EXERCISES.

The more difficult club exercises are not practicable in class drills. For this reason I introduce only a few of the more simple, such as can be easily adapted to music and used in classes. Such slow tunes as the Marseilles, are the best for exercises with the clubs.

The clubs for men, if made of hard wood, should be about eighteen inches long, and three or four inches in diameter. Women and children will adopt smaller ones. The floor should be so marked that the performers may, with certainty, occupy positions securing them against injuries from each other's clubs. If this be neglected a contusion of the knuckles, elbow, or head may greatly mar the pleasure of the lesson.

No. 1. The clubs hang at the sides, each hand grasping firmly, being careful not to push the index finger toward the body of the club, but keep it close with the rest of the hand. First raise the right arm as the left is represented in *Fig*. 1, five times. Same with the left. Then alternately and simultaneously, each five times.

Let it not be forgotten that in every exercise where it is possible, the right arm performs the feat first, then the left, then the two arms alternately, and last of all simultaneously. In each case the feat is to be executed five times. If the

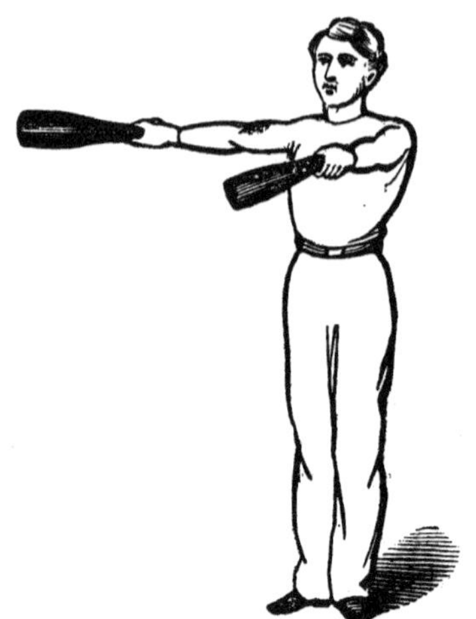

Figure 1.

teacher would make these exercises interesting and useful, he must insist upon the greatest accuracy. When the word of command is "*horizontal*," the club must be held *exactly* horizontal. When the word is "*perpendicular*," it should not vary from the perpendicular half an inch. In nearly all club exercises the arms must not be bent at the elbow. This point is very important, and very difficult to enforce.

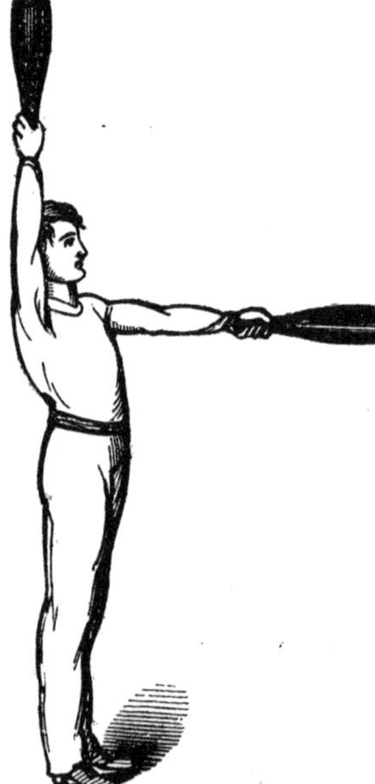

Figure 2.

No. 2. Raise the right arm and club as represented in *Fig*. 1. Left the same, etc.

No. 3. Holding the right

as the left is represented in *Fig.* 2, carry it directly upward until it is perpendicular. Left the same, etc.

No. 4. Holding the right as it is represented in *Fig.* 1, carry it directly upward sidewise until it is perpendicular. Left the same. etc.

No. 5. Right club should hang by the right leg. Carry it upward directly *in front*, until it is perpendicular over the shoulder. Left the same, etc.

No. 6. Right club hang by the side of the right leg. Carry it directly upward *sidewise* until perpendicular over the shoulder. Left the same, etc.

No. 7. Perform the right arm exercise of No. 2, and the left of No. 1, alternately and simultaneously.

No. 8. Execute the right of No. 3, and the left of No. 2, alternately and simultaneously.

No. 9. The right of No. 4, and the left of No. 3, alternately and simultaneously.

No. 10. The right of No. 5, and the left of No. 4, alternately and simultaneously.

No. 11. The right of No. 6, and the left of No. 5, alternately and simultaneously.

No. 12. Hold the two clubs as the left is represented in *Fig.* 2, without moving the arms, but simply by bending the wrist, and with a slow motion lay the right club down on its own arm. As it is carried back bring the left one down, and then work the two simultaneously.

No. 13. Hold the arms horizontal at the sides, as the right arm is shown in *Fig* 1, and execute the same exercise as in No. 12.

No. 14. Holding the two arms horizontal in front, and the clubs perpendicular, let the clubs fall sidewise, both to the right, until they are horizontal; then to the left, and so alternate five times. Now let them fall toward each other, then from each other, and so alternate five times.

No. 15. Hold the arms horizontal at the sides, and execute the same exercise as in No. 14.

No. 16. Arms horizontal in front, clubs perpendicular. Now carry the two arms in the horizontal plane,

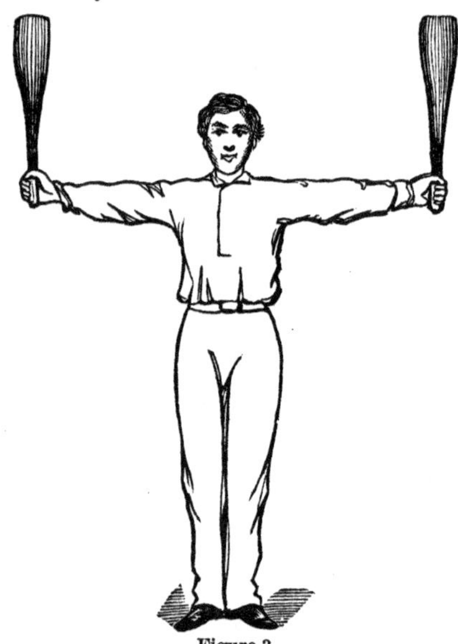

Figure 3.

without bending the elbows, backward as far as possible. (*Fig*. 3.) Halting touch the farther ends of the clubs on the back of the neck. Carry them out again to the position seen in *Fig*. 3. Now let the farther ends of the clubs touch at the nose. Carry them back again to *Fig*. 3 position. Let them fall backward, so that they hang down vertically, (*Fig*. 4.) but without moving the arms other than with a twisting motion. In this the hands must not be allowed to give way on

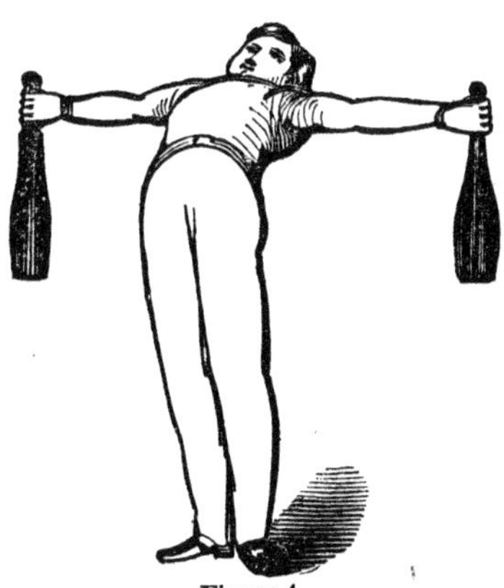

Figure 4.

the handle, but must grasp firmly. To reach this vertical position of the clubs as they fall behind, it is necessary to bend the back considerably. Raise the clubs again to *Fig*. 3 position, and allow them to fall again, but this time forward, and until they reach the vertical position. Thus alternate between the fall backward and forward, five times, and end by bringing the clubs to the hanging position by the side of the legs.

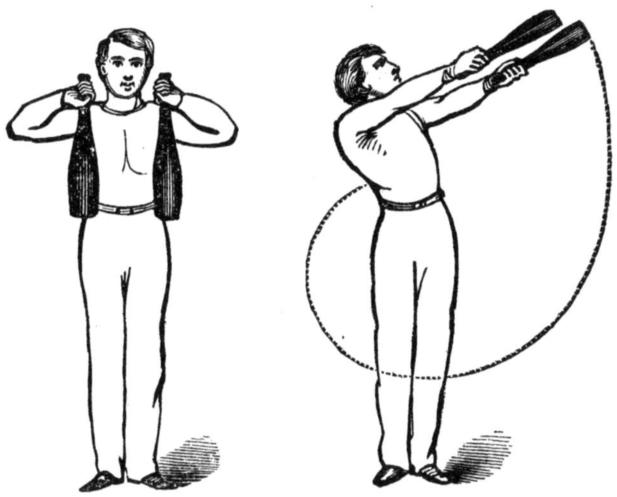

Figure 5. Figure 6.

No. 17. Hold the clubs as represented in *Fig*. 5. Carry their farther ends directly upward as far as you can reach them, and let them fall behind upon the shoulder blades. Thus alternate five times, or, if you please, fifty times.

No. 18. Hold the clubs as represented in *Fig*. 5, except they should be the other end up. Push the right one directly off the shoulder backward, and bringing it down by the side, raise it until it is horizontal in front. Now while this one is returning in the same track to the place of beginning, let the left one perform the same journey. And so alternate five times.

No. 19. Beginning as in No. 18, thrust the arms upwards and sidewise as seen in *Fig*. 6, and bringing them close down by the legs in front, carry them completely around the back, letting them fall down as far as possible and bring them to the chest, in the beginning position; thrust them up and out on the other side of the body, and carry them around the body the other way. Alternate five times.

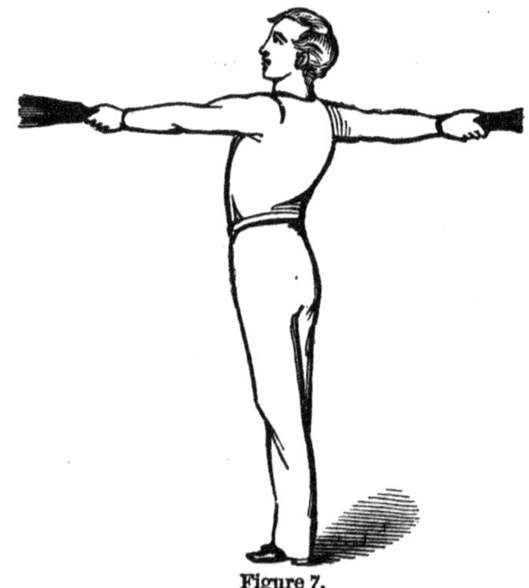

Figure 7.

No. 20. Holding the clubs as represented in *Fig.* 7, one exactly in front, the other behind, and both horizontal; carry them directly upward, and as they pass each other over the head they should be not more than one foot apart. Upon reaching the horizontal, the clubs, as will be seen, are exactly reversed. Be careful in this exercise not to bend the elbows or wrists.

Continue five times.

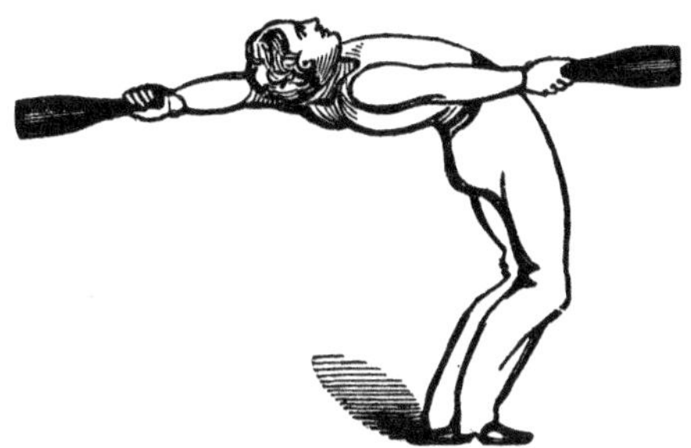

Figure 8.

No. 21. Holding the body, arms and clubs, as seen in *Fig.* 8, reverse the arms five times. If elbows or wrists be bent the exercise is lost.

No. 22. Holding the right club as represented in *Fig.* 2, and letting the left hang by the side, whirl the right slowly, in the horizontal plane, keeping the elbow and wrist quite stiff, (as in nearly all the other exercises,) and make a perfect circle with the farther end of the club. Then the same with the left. Alternately and simultaneously. The whirling in all the above is forward.

Now go over the same, whirling the club backward. Then whirl, with the same changes in front of the body, and lastly behind the back.

Pin Running.

One of the most exciting games ever devised, is one which, for want of a better name, I have christened *Pin Running*.

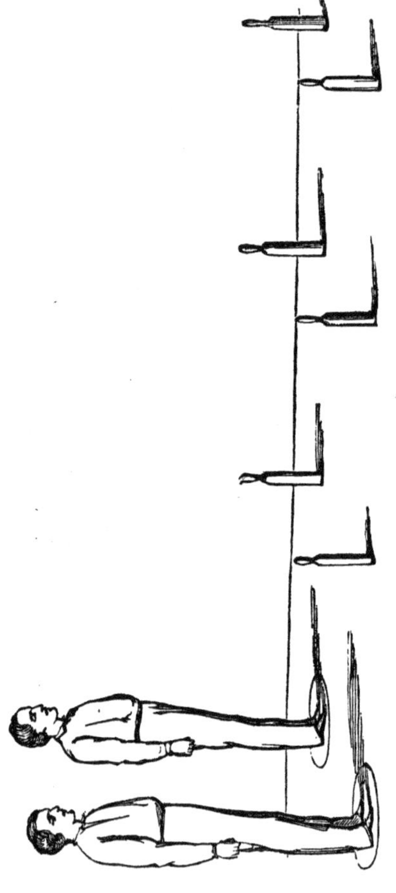

An examination of the cut will give a pretty good idea of the preparations for the game.

Three pins (ordinary clubs of the gymnasium) are placed on marks, which may be made with chalk, except in the case of a regular gymnasium, where they should be painted on the floor, in black or white.—The marks for each row of pins should be made in a straight line, at 15, 30 and 45 feet, respectively, from the centre of the goal. While these are the best distances, the size of the room may suggest or compel the adoption of another scale.

The goal in which each runner stands, is a circle of

two feet in diameter. The leader counts one, two, THREE, and each runner leaps to the first pin, which he hurries back and sets in the ring; then the second, and then the third. He who gets the third pin into the ring, and *has the three all standing*, *first*, is the victor, and counts one in the game.

The mode of procedure in this gymnasium, is to elect by nomination and acclamation two captains, who "choose sides," when the two parties contend in couples, and the tally is kept by setting up clubs in some conspicuous place, so that the members of both parties may know by a glance how the game stands.

Instead of having two rows of pins with two runners, three, four, or more may run at the same time, if the hall is wide enough.

There are numerous variations of this game, which will occur to every one.

For example, instead of the third pin, a bag of beans, weighing from twenty to fifty pounds, may be substituted, or a small boy may serve. And the rule, that the bag or boy shall be lifted and borne on the shoulder, may be adopted. But it will be found a very severe exercise. And even with the pins alone, the first few efforts will make the runners very lame. No person should run more than once on the first day. If in the enthusiasm this should be forgotten, a painful soreness will on the following day serve as a reminder.

A strong, swift runner may contend with a weak, slow one. The struggle in such a case may be made fair by omitting one of the pins in the row of the slow runner, or by adding one to that of the fast runner. In this way an interesting contest may be arranged between the two sexes, though the greatest speed I have ever witnessed, has been achieved by women.

Again, a vigorous man may contend with a delicate girl, he to use but one leg.

A hundred variations will suggest themselves to all who are interested.

Games with Birds' Nests.

This is a new kind of exercise, and a favorite in the gymnasium. It is cheap, easily put up, can be practiced without any instruction other than that I shall now give, and *tends to correct the habit of stooping*.

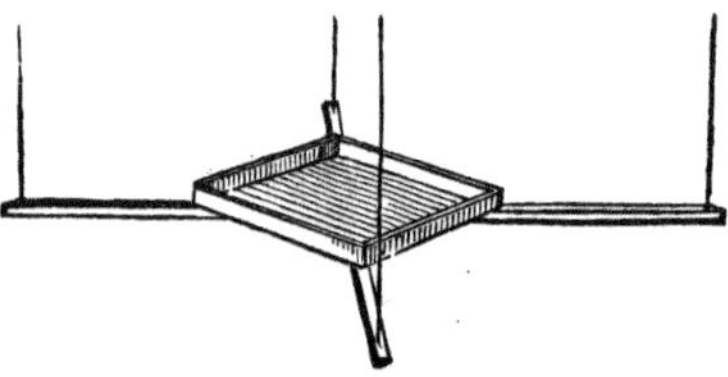

The above is a good representation of the nest. There should be four in the series, each of a different size. The ceiling of my gymnasium is eighteen feet from the floor. The room is sixty-five feet long. The ceiling lengthwise, I divided into four equal parts, and at these points I have hung the nests. The nests are square, measuring respectively 24, 18, 12 and 8 inches on a side; and the arms of each project one foot beyond the corners. The largest nest I have hung sixty inches from the ceiling; the next one forty inches; the third twenty inches; and the smallest one twelve inches. One of the cords supporting the nest, is in each case made to run through a pulley, and then to the side of the room, so that with the hand the nest may be tipped over and the bags thrown down. Now you are ready for the game. Holding a bag of beans, weighing three or four pounds, in both hands, under the chin, throw it upon the largest nest, and it counts one; throw it on the next one, and it counts two; on the third, which counts three; and on the fourth or smallest one, which counts four. Following one another in regular order, twenty or thirty persons may simultaneously engage in the game. It will readily occur to the reader that the bag may be thrown with the right hand alone, *always from the shoulder*, (never tossed,) then with the left. Then turning back toward the nest, toss the bag upon the nests over the head backward, though this is less profitable than those efforts in which you stand facing the nests.

The Arm Pull.

It is best to make it of rope, one-fourth of an inch in diameter, and two feet long, with perfect handles, so the hand will not get hurt, and very strong, so as to make certain that it shall never give way. A break that should allow some one to fall heavily on the floor, would be an unhappy affair.

Boys break their legs while coasting, or break through the ice and drown while skating, but no objection is made to coasting and skating. A slight accident in the gymnasium, and a cry of condemnation is heard on every hand. This is not strange; the gymnasium is comparatively new to our people. Teachers and managers must be exceedingly cautious.

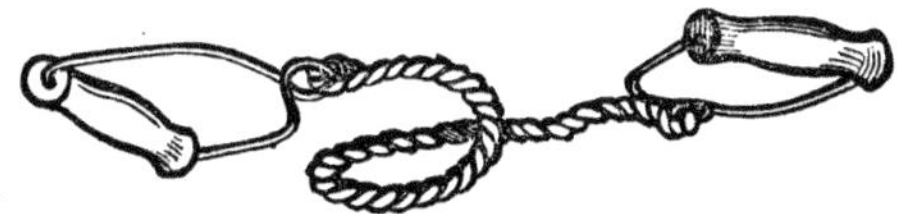

EXERCISES WITH THE ARM PULL.

No. 1. Use only one Pull in this exercise. Take hold of the handle with the right hand. Stand as far from your companion as possible, turn your right side toward him, and now, separating your legs wide, so that you may not tip over easily, draw upon your companion hard, but without moving your feet. As in his turn he does the same thing, you must give way without moving your feet. So you continue to draw to and fro, bending always sidewise.

No. 2. Left arm the same.

No. 3 Using two Pulls you face each other, and each holds with the right hand the Pull held with the other's left. Draw backward and forward alternately, twenty or thirty times.

In this and in Nos. 4, 5 and 6, when your right arm goes forward, the left is drawn backward.

No. 4. Same as the last, except that the Pulls do not cross between you, so that the Pull held with the right hand of one, is held with the right hand of the other, and your left hands take hold of the same Pull. Now draw backward and forward alternately, twenty or thirty times.

No. 5. Standing your backs to each other, connect your hands with the two Pulls, and draw backward and forward as far as you can move the hands.

No. 6. Same as the last, except that your backs are allowed to touch each other.

Each "Pull" should cost 25 cents.

In speaking of the cost of this and some other pieces of apparatus, I simply desire to give the manufacturer and buyer a guide. The prices are those I have been obliged to pay,

GYMNASTIC CROWN.

Bearing burthens on the head, results in an erect spine and an elastic gait. Observing persons, who have visited Switzerland, Italy, or the Gulf States, have observed a thousand verifications of this physiological law.

Cognizant of the value of this feature of gymnastic training, I have employed, for this purpose, within the last twelve years, various sorts of weights, but have recently invented an iron crown, which I think completely satisfactory. The accompanying cut gives a good idea of its general form. I have them made to weigh from three to one hundred pounds. The crown is so padded within, it rests pleasantly on the entire top of the head, and yet so arranged that it requires skill to balance it. It is beautifully painted, and otherwise ornamented.

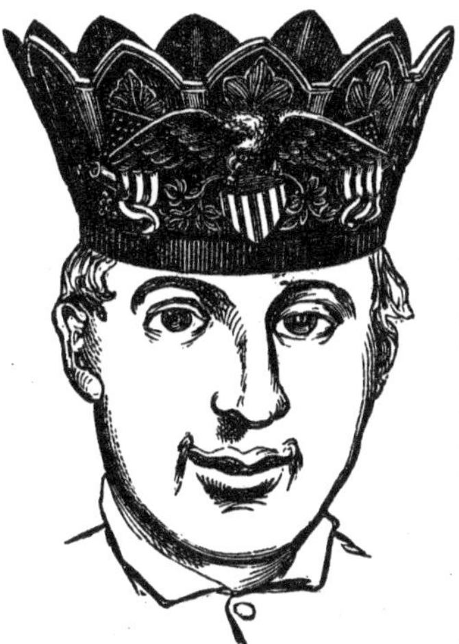

THE FOLLOWING SUGGESTIONS are deemed important in wearing the crown:—Wear it five to fifteen minutes morning and evening. Hold the body erect, hips and shoulders thrown far back, and the crown rather on the front of the head, as shown in the cut.

Walking up and down stairs while wearing the crown, is good, if the lower extremities are not too much fatigued by it. When walking through the hall or parlors, turn the toes, first, inward as far as possible; second, outward; third, walk on the tips of the toes; fourth, on the heels; fifth, on the right heel and left toe; sixth, on the left heel and right toe; seventh, walk without bending the knees; eighth, bend the knees, so that you are nearly sitting on the heels while walking, ninth, walk with the right leg bent at the knee, rising at each step on the straight left leg; tenth, walk with the left leg bent, rising at each step on the straight right leg.

With these ten different modes of walking, the various muscles of the back will receive the most invigorating exercise.

All persons of both sexes, and of every age, who have round shoulders or weak backs, are rapidly improved by the use of the Gymnastic Crown.

The Shoulder Pusher.

The arm pieces should be seven inches long and of the shape represented in the cut, and so rounded as not to hurt the shoulders, and made so blunt and round

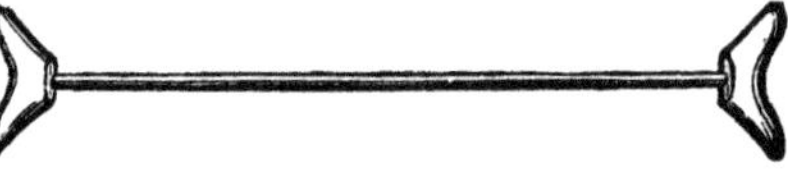

at the points, that ladies shall not suffer an injury in the breast by an unlucky slip.

The connecting rod should be two and a half feet long, and one inch and a half thick, of ash, and put into the handles very strong, so that it cannot break, and tear the shoulders with a sharp point. I have never known an accident to occur with them, but if the instrument were badly made, can imagine it possible.

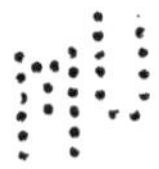

Every thing should be polished, so that no little sliver can scratch the hand.

EXERCISES.—In all the exercises with the Shoulder Pusher, the party must be divided into couples, as two are necessary to each exercise.

No. 1. In this exercise one pusher only is used. Each puts his right shoulder against the arm piece, and in this position you push each other.

No. 2. The same with the left shoulder.

No. 3. Use two pushers, and putting the shoulders against the arm pieces, standing face to face, push as hard as you please.

No. 4. Use one pusher, placing it against the right arm at the elbow; your friend the same. Push hard.

No. 5. Left the same.

No. 6. Then with two pushers, simultaneously.

No. 7. Using only the right arm, place the hand against the arm piece, and extending the arm toward your friend, horizontally and at full length, push hard. Now, sinking almost to your knees, while your friend rises to his toes, push again. Then he sinks while you rise, and you push again. Then you step one foot to the right, while your friend steps one foot to his right, and remaining in this position, go through with the same exercises as when you were standing face to face. Now step one foot to the left, your friend to his left, and repeat the same exercises.

No. 8. Same with the left hand.

No. 9. Same with both hands.

Some of these exercises are difficult, but they secure the play of certain muscles that are not moved in the same manner by any other exercise.

Each "Pusher" should cost 25 cents.

FREE GYMNASTICS.

The word "*free*," is used in this connection as indicating those exercises in which no apparatus is employed. They are profitable and happily adapted to the school room; but some object in the hand will add greatly to the *interest* and profit of gymnastic training.

The teacher may invent a new series occasionally to keep up the interest. Since I began to teach gymnastics I have invented and used an immense number of free gymnastics.

The following, devised by the distinguished SCHREBER, are given as samples, by way of suggestion.

These exercises should all be performed to music.

In devising new exercises, it is necessary to keep in mind one or two points. First, the exercises should tend directly to force the shoulders backward, and open the chest. Second, the neck, sides and back should have varied and vigorous training.

Rolling Head Movement, (Fig. 1.)

Five times from right to left, and five times from left to right.

Sidewise Head Movement, (Fig. 2.)

Five times each way.

These two movements are good to strengthen the muscles of the neck, and are remedial in a case of ver-

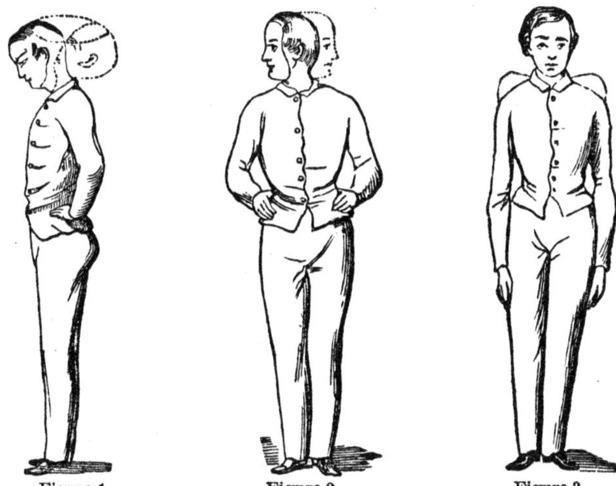

Figure 1. Figure 2. Figure 3.

tigo. When first using these, the motions must be very slow.

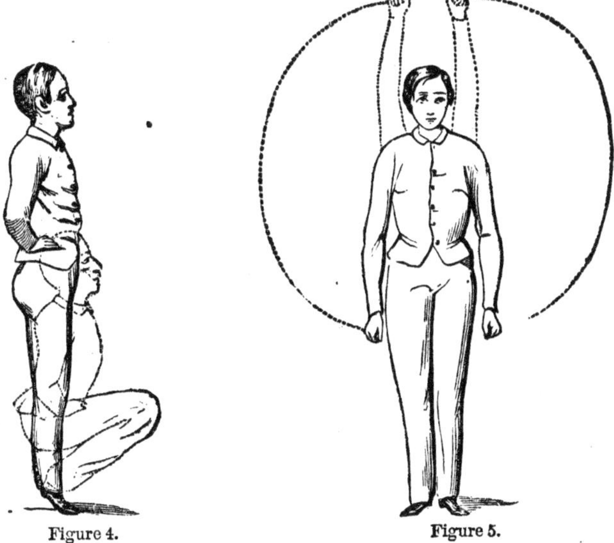

Figure 4. Figure 5.

Shoulder Lifting, (Fig. 3.)

First raise the right shoulder as high as possible, then the left, alternately and simultaneously, each ten times, keeping heels together and shoulders back. I would add here that the shoulders and heels must be kept in these positions in all the exercises, where it is possible.

Sinking and Raising the body, (Fig. 4.)

Sink down till you touch the heels, and then rise to your utmost height twenty times. Most capital exercise; especially in dyspepsia and constipation.

Raising the Arms Sidewise, (Fig. 5.)

The arms are to be carried from the sides to the perpendicular position over the shoulders and down again, twenty times. In this and all the other exercises the

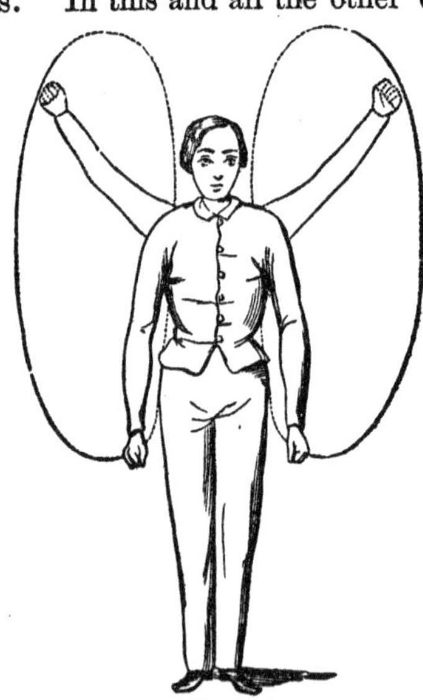

Figure 6.

teacher must be very particular in regard to the position of his pupils—*heels togeτner, shoulders drawn far back.*

Circular Arm Movement, (Fig. 6.)

Right hand held perpendicularly over the shoulder, dashes *forward*, and is whirled round and round, coming to rest by the side. Left arm the same. Alternately and simultaneously the same, each ten times. Again raise the right arm, dash it *backward*, and whirl it round and round. Left arm the same. Alternately and simultaneously the same, each ten times.

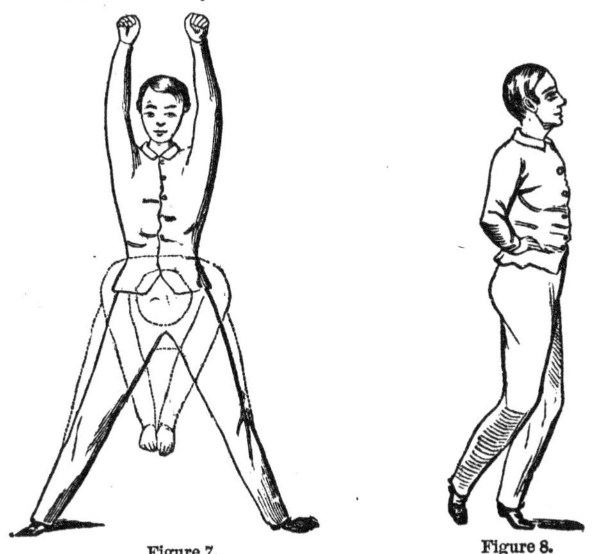

Figure 7. Figure 8.

Chopping Movement, (Fig. 7.)

Ten times up and down.

Trotting Movement, (Fig. 8.)

Stand still in one spot and hop a few inches from the floor on one foot. Then the other foot. Alternately and simultaneously, each twenty times.

Sawing Movement, (Fig. 9.)

Thrust each hand forward and downward, at the

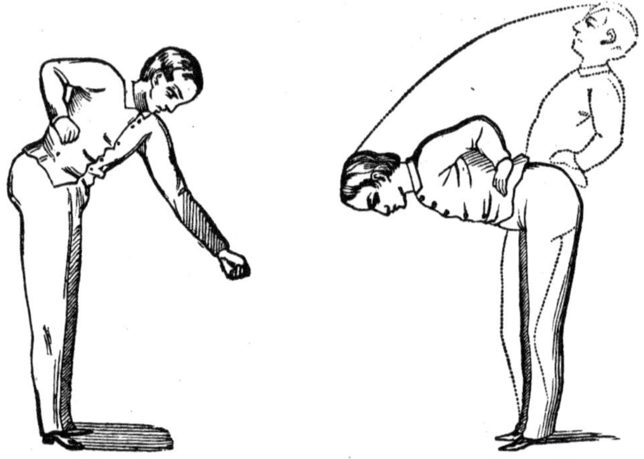

Figure 9. Figure 10.

same time drawing the elbow of the other arm backward as far as possible, twenty times. Most excellent exercise.

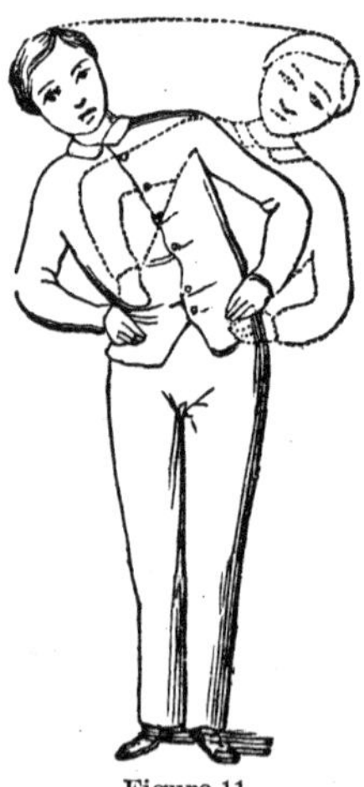

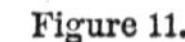

Figure 11.

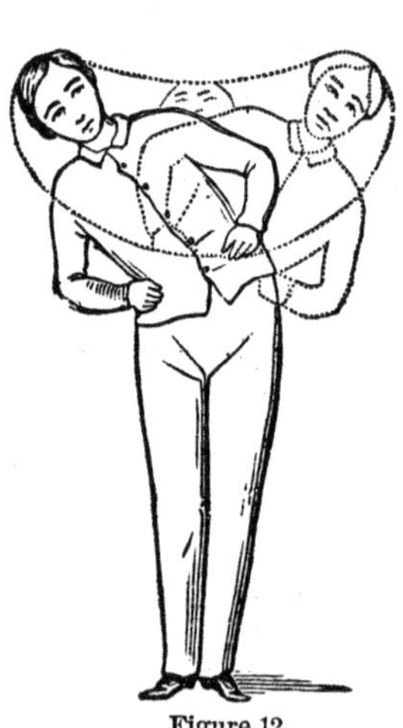

Figure 12.

Bending the Body Forward and Backward, (Fig. 10.)
Move the body very slowly each way, ten times.

Sideward Movement of the Body, (Fig. 11.)
Move from side to side slowly, ten times.

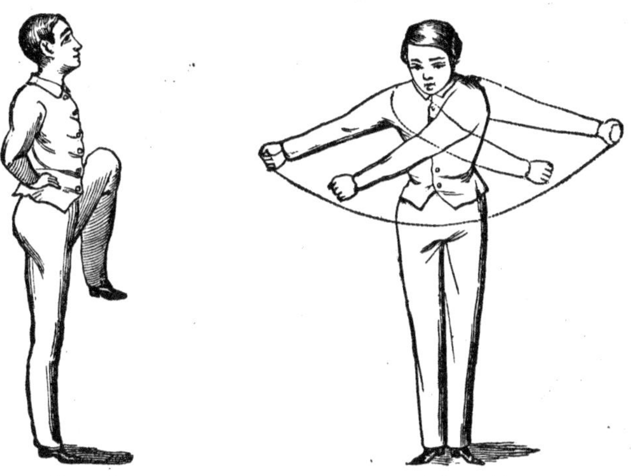

Figure 13. Figure 14.

Twisting of the Body, (Fig. 12.)
Twist the body each way, ten times. Splendid for bad livers, and very bad for tight dresses.

Raising the Knee, (Fig. 13.)
Raise each knee as high as you can, ten times.

Swinging Arms Sidewise, (Fig. 14.)
Swing each way twenty times, as hard as you can, without moving the feet.

Swinging the Arms Apart, (Fig. 15.)
With force backward, twenty times.

Swinging the Leg Sidewise, (Fig. 16.)
Both ways, as far as possible, in front of the other

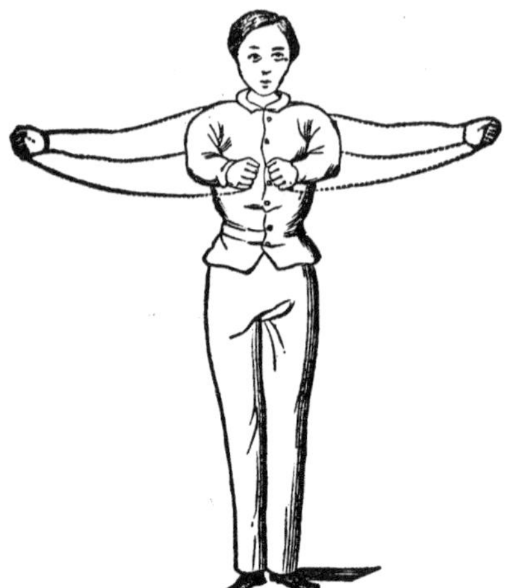

Figure 15.

leg, tweuty times. Then behind the other leg, as far as possible, twenty times.

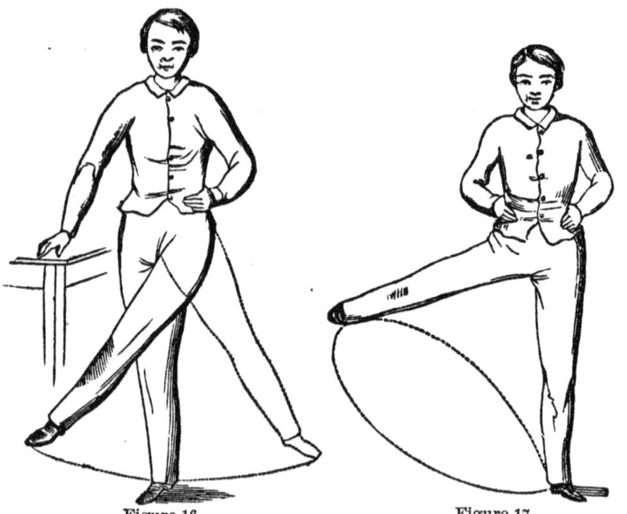

Figure 16. Figure 17.

Circular Movement of the Leg, (Fig. 17.) Each leg in both directions, twenty times.

Stretching the Arms Downward, Behind, (Fig. 18.)
With force, but slowly, twenty times.

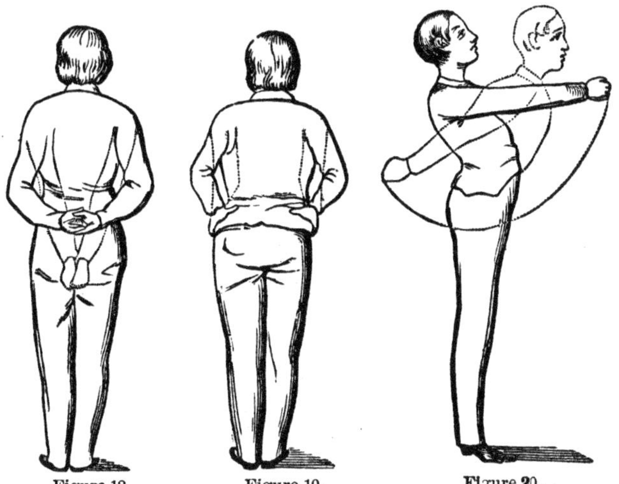

Figure 18. Figure 19. Figure 20.

Throwing back the Elbows, (Fig. 19.)
With force, but very slowly, ten times.

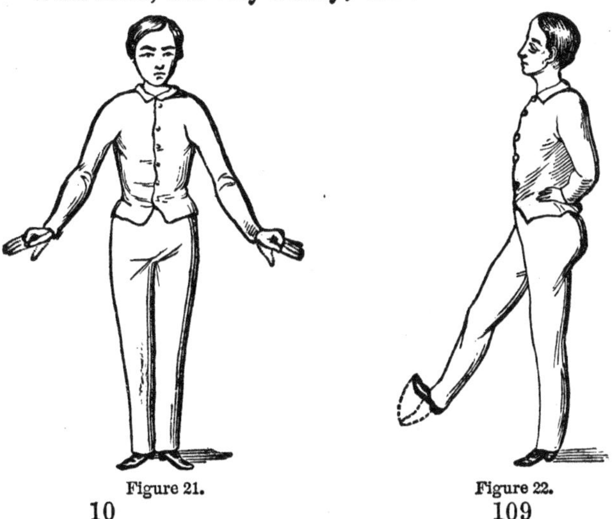

Figure 21. Figure 22.

Swinging the Arms Backward and Forward, (Fig. 20.)

In precisely the manner represented, swing the arms thirty times.

Opening and Shutting the Hands, (Fig. 21.)

The hands to be opened and shut as indicated, with force, twenty times.

Bending and Stretching the Foot, (Fig. 22.)

First raise and depress the toe, ten times. Then make a large and complete circle with the toe, ten times.

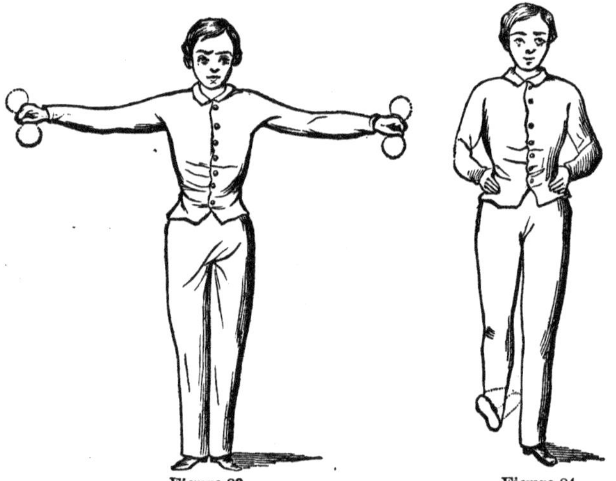

Figure 23. Figure 24.

Fig. Eight Movement of the Hands, (Fig. 23.)

Move the hands, closed as represented, describing the figure (∞) horizontally.

Twisting the Legs, (Fig. 24.)

Holding the ankle stiff, twist the whole leg so that the toe moves from right to left as far as possible, ten times.

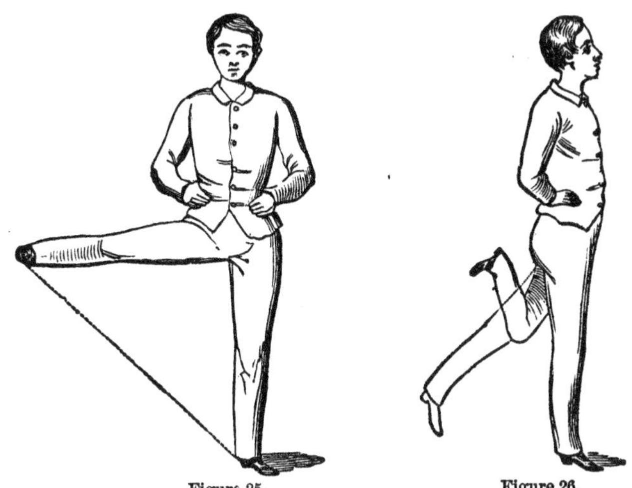

Figure 25. Figure 26.

Sideward Movement of the Leg, (Fig. 25.)
Each foot fifteen times.

Bending and Stretching the Leg Behind, (Fig. 26.)
Each leg twenty times.

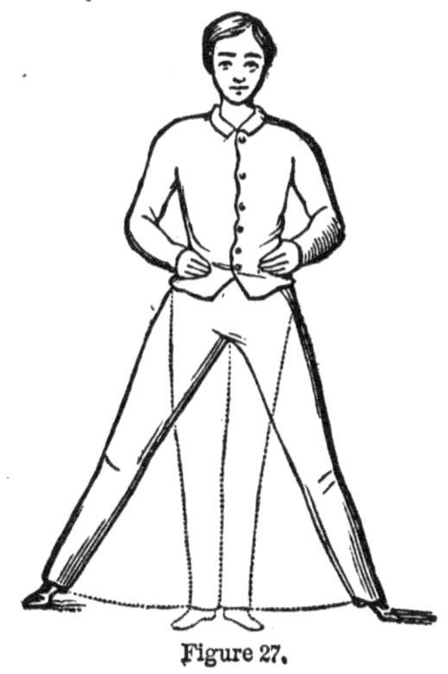

Figure 27.

Legs Out and Back Sidewise, (Fig. 27.)

With spirit and force, twenty times.

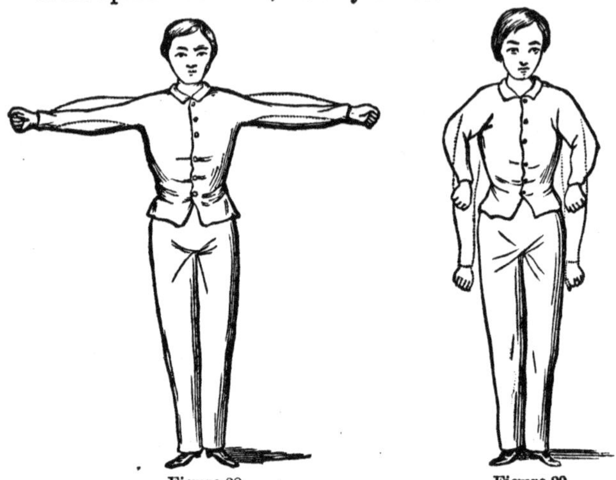

Figure 28. Figure 29.

Twisting the Arms, (Fig. 28.)

Holding the hands horizontal, twist the arms backward and forward, ten times each way.

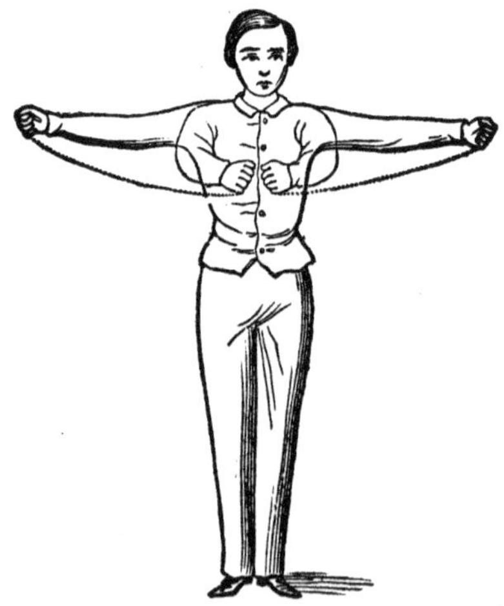

Figure 30.

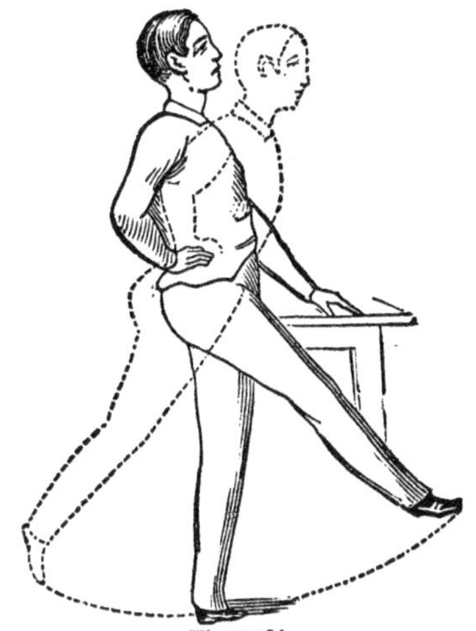

Figure 31.

Striking the Hands Downward, (Fig. 29.)
Twenty times with great force.

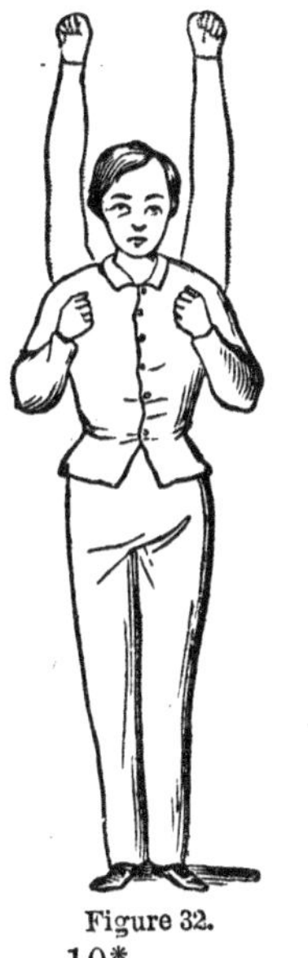

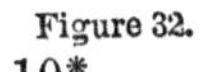

Figure 32.

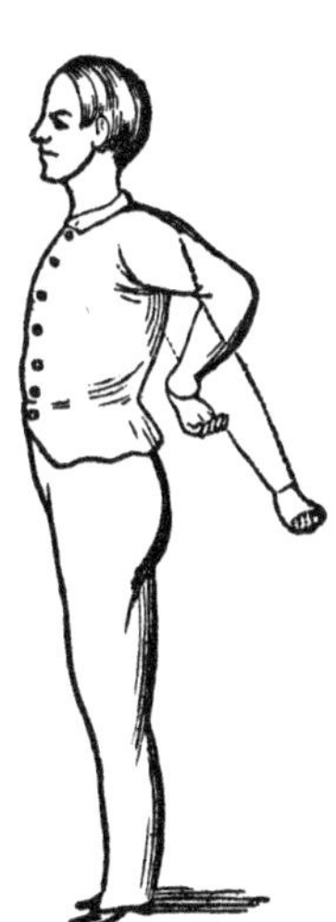

Figure 33.

Swinging the Arms together, (Fig. 30.)

Carry them backward slowly, and bring them forward with force, twenty times.

Swing the Leg Backward and Forward, (Fig. 31.)

Study the cut carefully, and perform the movement, ten times.

Hands Upward, (Fig. 32.)

Perpendicularly thirty times.

Hands Backward, (Fig. 33.)

With force, ten times.

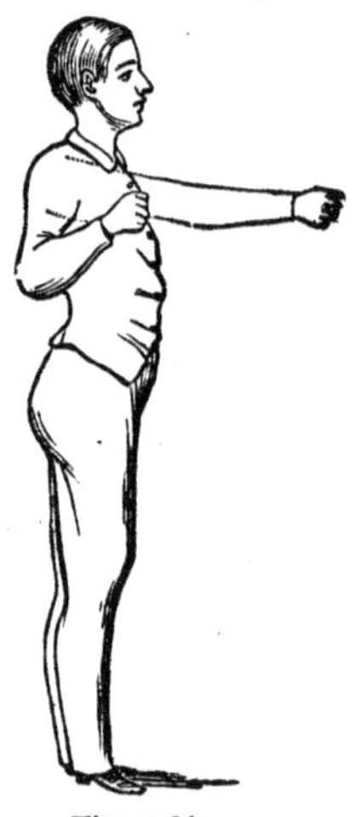

Figure 34.

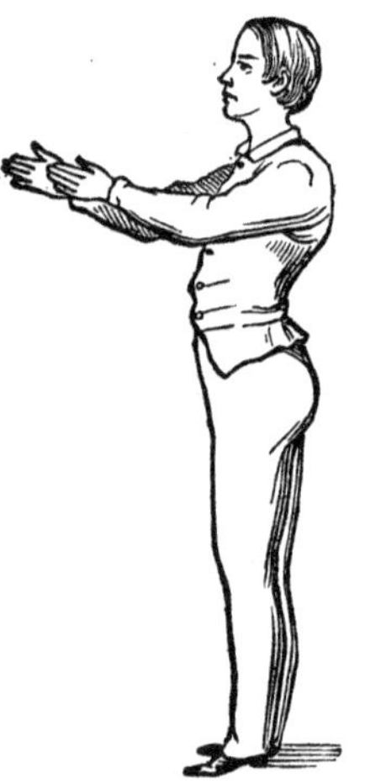

Figure 35.

Hands alternately Forward, (Fig. 34.)

Each hand with great energy, twenty-five times.

Rubbing the Hands together without Bending the Elbows, (Fig. 35.)

If the hands are drawn completely by each other, it will be found a most capital exercise for the shoulders. Indeed, but few persons can perform the feat at all, at first.

Count only the right hand and draw it backward, thirty times.

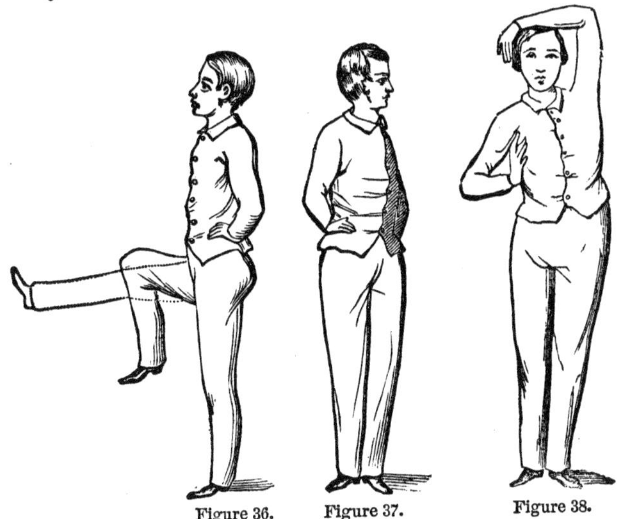

Figure 36. Figure 37. Figure 38.

Bending and Stretching the Leg Forward, (Fig. 36.) Twenty times, as indicated in the cut.

Twisting the Body, [Fig. 37.]

Don't move the feet, and twist the body, holding the hands on the sides, and keeping the shoulders back as far as possible, *fifty times*, quite slow.

Deep Breathing with Body Bent Sidewise, [Fig. 38.] Bend the body sidewise as far as possible, with the hands in the position seen in the cut, and take five deep breaths. Of course in all these exercises both sides are to receive the same treatment.

THE

DUMB BELL INSTRUCTOR

FOR

PARLOR GYMNASTS.

AN ACCESSION TO PRACTICAL PHYSIOLOGY,

BY

PROFESSOR MAURICE KLOSS,

Director of the Royal Saxon Normal Gymnastic Institute in Dresden.

With 20 Illustrations.

THIRD EDITION.

Translated from the German, by

DIO LEWIS, M. D.,

and published in this work as an important addition to the New Dumb Bell Exercises.

"The solution of the great and important problem, the comprehension of which will deliver the greater portion of the Human family from the dominion of disease, and permit them to enjoy life to the utmost length, and health to the utmost extent, permitted by Nature—the utility to strengthen every organ of the physical system, and supply it with the greatest power of resistance against all external influences:—ALL THIS is contained in the single word GYMNASTICS."

DR. K. W. IDELER, Medical Counsellor,
Professor of Physiology, &c., in Berlin.

PREFACE. *

Man's physical integrity must ever depend upon his fidelity to nature. Through the deteriorating influences of civilization, he has departed far from nature. If he would restore his life-energy, he must, like the prodigal son, return.

Health is the most precious of earthly possessions. He who has it, has all things; he who lacks it, has nothing. Men seek with vehement earnestness, external things. How few recognize the value of health. Men seem to care as little for their bodies as the snail for its shell. The world is full of misery. Physical deformity and suffering are increasing with fearful rapidity. Thank God, the great physiological revolution which is to restore man to his pristine condition, has been inaugurated.

As in the prosecution of all other reforms, we are met on every hand by prejudice. We are told that man was not designed to enjoy uninterrupted health; that in this life he must be the victim of disease and suffering; that nature will give all needed superinten-

* In justice to Prof. KLOSS, I should state, that in translating this little work, I have taken the utmost liberty with the original. In some cases an entire page has been compressed into a single, brief paragraph. I intended at first to publish a literal translation, but when I had finished, and read it to several intelligent friends, they unanimously advised me to re-write it, adapting it to the American mind. This has been done, but without essential alterations in the ideas of the author.

The descriptions of the various exercises, and what is said of the weight of the Dumb Bells, are all faithful translations.—*Translator.*

dence to the body. True, they say, it is possible to ward off danger, but quite chimerical to undertake the prevention of disease by a development of the powers within. Hufeland took this view of the subject. But the physiological reformer of the present hour affirms that the physical organism is susceptible of indefinite improvement; that it can be made, by certain hygienic processes, so vigorous and resistant, that amid diseases and dangers it may pass through the fire unscathed.

How shall such invigoration of our bodies be secured? So far as the answer can be given in one word, it is *gymnastics*. In the animal body, exercise is the principal law of development. By gymnastics, we mean a system of exercises which the greatest wisdom and largest experience have devised, as best adapted to the complete development of the physical man. IDELER was the first to comprehend the principles of gymnastics, and their application to the training of the body. He saw their infinite worth in the education of youth; in the preservation of the health of adults; and in the cure of many diseases.

Gymnastics are valuable to all persons, but especially to clerks, students, sedentary artisans, and still more particularly, to those who in addition to sedentary habits, perform exhaustive intellectual labor. With the latter class, suffering from indigestion and nervous irritability, nothing but a wise system of gymnastic training can prevent the early failure of the powers of life. We believe that to such persons this little work will come as a most welcome friend. We believe that it may assist them in returning to health and nature. Do not, friends, we implore you, refuse its kind offices by such pleas as "want of time," the "great difficulty of the feats," "age," "rigidity of limbs," or "want of strength;" for if these excuses are well founded in your case, the exercises described in this little work, will prove to you of great value.

The reader will find descriptions and illustrations of a large number of the most valuable exercises with dumb bells. The descriptions are so simple that there will be no difficulty in understanding them.

It is hoped that in this little book many persons will find a simple means, through which they may secure a full use of all their powers. May they find in it a source of health and happiness.

M. KLOSS.

DRESDEN, MAY, 1860.

DUMB BELL INSTRUCTOR.

CHAPTER I.

History and Use of Dumb Bells.

The intellectual progress of nations and individuals, depends greatly upon their physical vigor. The ancient Greeks understood this and well expressed it in the thought: "a healthy soul can live only in a healthy body." Nor did they content themselves by merely expressing this thought in words, as their elaborated system of gymnastic training demonstrates. They knew that thorough gymnastic culture made *whole men;* fitting them for the pursuits of war or peace, science or art. Greek gymnastics gave strength, grace and agility. It intermarried soul and body. Their statesmen, warriors, artists, and men of science, challenge our admiration. They respected the laws of health and became vigorous. We heed them not; hence modern physical decline. By our artificial modes of life, we are losing all taste for that which we most need. Because of this distaste for bodily exercise, we have adopted a one-sided system of culture, which leaves the body entirely out of view, and which works upon it in a destructive manner. We must seek restoration mainly through efficient physical training. For this, we look to the gymnasium. The modern gymnasium is without doubt superior to that of the Greeks, yet because it is not generally established, or because those who most need its training, consider themselves too weak, or aged, or awkward; or because in our institutions of learning, body-culture is not thought of, few realize the benefits of a thorough gymnastic education.

The little dumb bell should remind us of the gymnastic palaces of the Greeks. To them, as well as to other very ancient nations, its use and value were well known. By means of it we wish to popularize modern gymnastics.

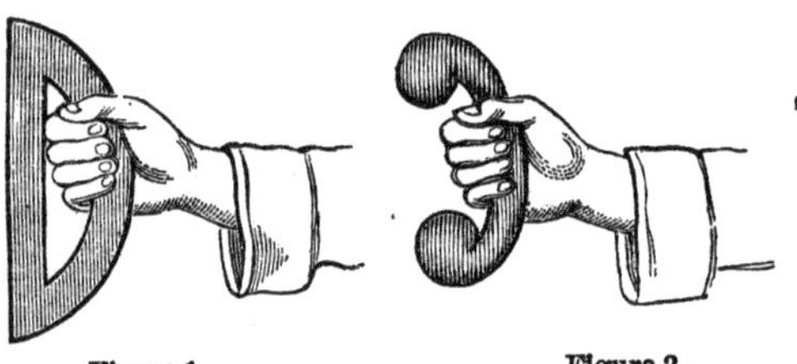

Figure 1. Figure 2.

Its shape, as first used by the Greeks is seen in *Fig.* 1. Their improved bell was much like that in use at the present time. *(Fig. 2.)* These dumb bells were made of lead and were taken in both hands to serve as a balance or support in those springing exercises which the Greeks held to be of great value.

Besides being used in these leaping exercises, they were employed, as by us, in a great variety of ways, for strengthening the muscles of the arms and chest. Aristotle, Seneca, and other ancient writers, speak of their uses and value. Martial and Juvenal mention even women who used them with facility.

The discovery of representations of the dumb bell, upon ancient Grecian earthern vessels, led to their introduction into England, where their use became very general. Their simplicity, cheapness and adaptation to home-use, have rendered them popular in Great Britain.

Those introduced from India, which were for a time much used, are not adapted to moderate sized rooms, on account of their length.

Cast iron dumb bells are now most in use. They should be of equal weight and adapted to the strength of the pupil. For women and children they should weigh from two to three pounds; for male adults from two to five pounds.

Dumb bells weighing three pounds are sufficiently heavy for producing thorough exercise of the body, in the strongest man; those weighing more, though they call out greater exertion, will prevent that active exercise which is most valuable. Bells weighing fifty and one hundred pounds are serviceable only in trials of strength; by their frequent use a one-sided condition is produced.

Few persons can enjoy the advantages of a gymnasium, but with this book, and with the dumb bells, its benefits can be secured at home by Parlor Gymnastics.

Those accustomed to walk for exercise will find that the dumb bell, properly managed, will not only save time, but prove a more efficient means of bringing every muscle of the body into vigorous action. So valuable are they considered that in many armies they are used in addition to the drill, to secure a more thorough development of the soldiers. In all exercises with them perfect time should be observed.

CHAPTER II.

Important Rules applicable to the Practice of Dumb Bell Exercises.

The good results which follow gymnastic exercises, depend entirely upon their correct application; therefore we present some general suggestions with reference to dumb bell exercises.

Heavy garments, and those so close fitting as to prevent a free motion of every part of the body, should be removed.

In commencing the exercises, be gentle, and increase their vigor and duration as the body becomes capable of bearing them. Muscular development is secured by the operation of natural laws, and sudden or excessive exertion interferes with these laws and produces harm.

Be satisfied with a small advance daily; in this way only, can improvement be made certain. Those, who, for want of exercise, have become debilitated, must not think that by the violent use of dumb bells they can make up for lost time, or immediately become strong; with such a course, they will be likely to reach exactly opposite results, and become disgusted with gymnastic studies. Nature will not permit such transitions. No machine can suddenly be put in motion at its highest possible speed, and as suddenly stopped, without risk of destroying it. The body is more especially injured by such a course. Its nutrition, by which only it can be built up, is a slow process, and cannot by violent efforts be accelerated. When gymnastic exercises unfit one for his usual occupation, they fail in their object. It is easy to perceive the extent to which they may be carried, and to adapt them to the habits of life, by which means only can they prove a foundation for the security of health. Take time, therefore, to go through with the exercises in a manner most appropriate to the bodily conditions.

Avoid a sudden transition from one exertion to another. Do not engage in difficult dumb bell exercises immediately after fatiguing mental labor; or just before or after a hearty meal; for, then, the life-forces centre in the stomach, and if withdrawn to the muscles the process of digestion is disturbed.

Those who have much mental labor to perform, should avoid fatiguing exercises in the morning, as the diversion of nervous energy from the brain will render thinking more difficult. To such, easy exercises in the morning will drive away that languor which sometimes follows sleep, and prepare the person for active brain labor; while in the afternoon, which is not favorable to exhausting efforts of the mind, appropriate physical exercise may be taken. For some, ten minutes exercise with dumb bells, immediately after the morning ablution, produces a delightful glow, and excellent results; to others, an hour before dinner, or an hour before retiring, is found more advantageous. To all, there can, no doubt, be found an appropriate time when mental labor can be interrupted for that training which will secure strength, appetite and sleep, and preserve the body for a continuance of all that belongs to its external life.

The moderate temperature of spring and autumn serves to advance mental and physical vigor, and thorough exercise may then be taken. By natural instinct we may know that during the summer heat, physical labor should be moderate; yet those who are vigorous will find that the vital energies are increased by sufficient exercise in summer, provided it is not taken when the heat is excessive. Those who are effeminate may find it best to yield to inactivity at this season.

In winter, nutrition is most active, and the amount of exercise may be increased; but it should not be taken in a highly heated room. Active exercise of the muscles has always proved of great value in preparing the body to resist cold. Dr. Ideler says: "there is but one method of inuring the body to the action of cold, and that is to expose one's self to it during vigorous exercise."

Avoid sudden transitions from rest to great exertion, and the reverse. It is best to commence with light exercises, and arrange to have the most difficult ones come in the middle of the lesson.

It is important that a full supply of fresh air be secured, and frequently during the exercises it is advisable to take a long deep breath.

To secure an uniform distribution of the exercise over the body, it is necessary that each movement be pursued to the same extent, by each half of the body.

The frequency of the exercises must depend on each one's necessity. The eminent Dr. Ideler says: "it is not necessary that every organ be daily exerted to its greatest capacity. Our organism permits large scope in this respect. Were we to become bound in our gymnastic training to the exact mechanical swing of the pendulum, it would be impossible for us to fulfil the higher demands of our mental and social nature. For the student, one or two lessons in vigorous exercises each week will be sufficient. *Every organ when brought to its full tension has a tendeney to continue unimpaired for a long time.* Most of the infirmities of the higher classes, and of students, result from the neglect of gymnastic training, and the too excessive activity of the nervous system.

Persons advanced in years should confine themselves to those movements which do not greatly accelerate the circulation, or produce fatigue. Let them at first go through the exercises without the dumb bells. If slight soreness is produced, it will soon disappear. *By gradual steps, even the bodies of those growing old will become flexible and fresh.* Very young people should keep aloof from violent exertions. Let them commence with the easy exercises, and go on, step by step, to the difficult ones.

To the mature man beneficial effects will only follow through persevering exertions.

CHAPTER III.

Dumb Bell Exercises without change of position, with special reference to the Development of the Arms aud Upper portion of the body.

Pupils stand erect; head, shoulders and hips drawn well back; chest pressed forward; heels together; toes separated so that the feet form with each other a right angle.

In this position the characteristics of man are most distinctly marked. No other creature can walk so erect. Upon this attitude depends the usefulness of his senses, complete respiration, tone of his voice, and the highest uses of his arms and legs.

It is difficult to maintain this position for any considerable time. Nearly all the muscles of the body are brought into vigorous action by its maintenance, but more particularly those of the neck, spine, and shoulder blades. All the functions of the thoracic and abdominal viscera are favored by this position, while the circulation of the blood is accelerated. It follows that this erect carriage is exceedingly favorable to the health and vigor of man. How few men possess this noble bearing! Among women it is still more rare! Our dumb bell friends must keep before their minds the importance of this upright position. To those whose business compels a stooping posture, this advice is particularly important.

The best exercises of the upper half of the body must all rest upon the position we have described.—When the heels touch each other, with the toes so separated as to form a right angle, the feet are said to be in a *locked position*, and when the feet are separated they are spoken of as in an *apart position*.

A.

Arm Exercises with Dumb Bells.

The following exercises are adapted to music. When the time is double, it will be indicated by 2-2; treble, 3-3; quadruple, 4-4; and so on, 5-5, 6-6, 7-7, 8-8.

An exercise in 4-4 time, is one in which the movements are regulated by four even equi-distant counts, ONE, *two*, *three*, *four*. Some of the exercises are accented; *i. e.* on some one or more of the beats there is bestowed more force. If the accent is on the first count, the leader counts ONE, *two*, *three*, *four*. The movements of the dumb bells should correspond with the counting.

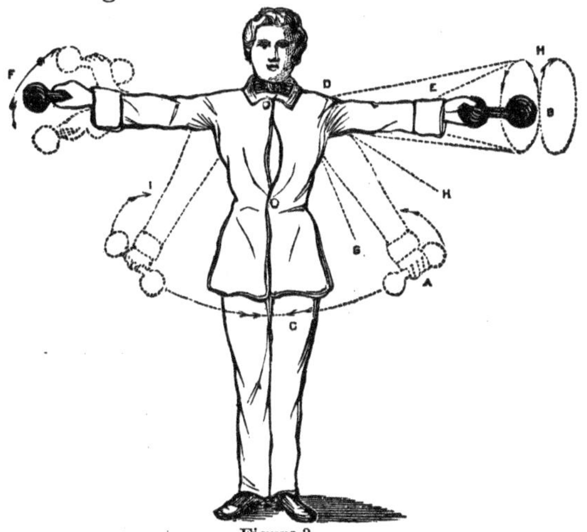

Figure 3.

When the hand grasps the bell, with the back of the hand upward, (*Fig.* 3, A,) it is called the *Wrist Grasp*; when with the palm up, it is known as the *Comb Grasp;* with the thumb upward, the *Spoke Grasp;* with the little finger upward, the *Ell Grasp*.

1. *First Exercise*. Arms hanging down as in *Fig.* 4, A, 4-4 time.

Count *one*, and carry arms out sideways, position *Fig.* 3, A.

Two: Arms down again.

Three: Lift the arms sideways to the horizontal position, as in *Fig.* 3, B.

Four: Arms down again by the sides.

At the will of the leader the movements may be alternated by *invertion*; *i. e.* the movement executed with the last count *four*, may be made with the count *one*. So the leader counts *One* on the 4th position.

Two " " 3d "

Three " " 2d "

Four " " 1st "

This exercise may be varied in the following manner:—

Count *one*, left arm sideways, to the obliquè position, (*Fig.* 3, G.)

Two, left arm sideways, to the oblique position, (*Fig.* 3, A.)

Three, left arm sideways, to the oblique position, (*Fig.* 3, H.)

Four, left arm sideways, to the horizontal position, (*Fig.* 3, B.)

In the same manner the arms are to be let down again. A still greater effort is required if at count *one*, the arms are raised to the horizontal position at once, and then gradually let down while counting two, three, four. In order that during the continuance of these simple exercises the legs may not remain entirely inactive, the pupil may add to the raising and lowering of the dumb bells, local walking; that is, walking without moving from his place. Every step is followed by one of the positions indicated in *Figs.* 3 and 4; the motions of the feet and those of the arms conforming to the time. The vigorous pupil may carry this to the running speed.

A further variation can be produced in this exercise by raising one arm, while the other is being lowered.

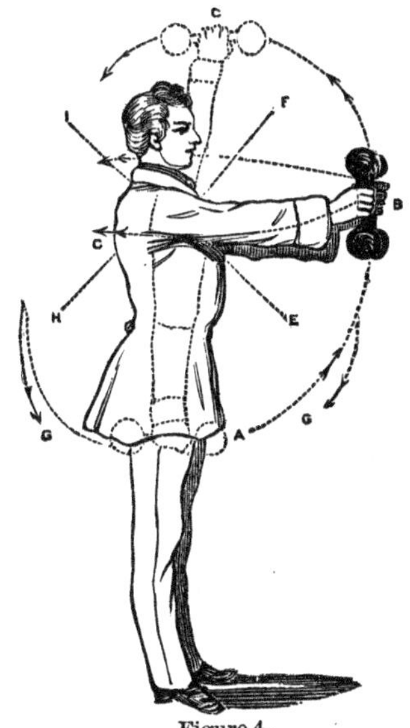

Figure 4.

A simple series of exercises is found in raising the arms in front, as seen in *Fig*. 4, instead of sideways as in *Fig*. 3; and, in this series, a larger scope may be reached by carrying the dumb bells above the horizontal position, (*Fig*. 4, B,) to the *point* position, (*Fig*. 4, C.) In this attitude the arms are held perpendicular, near the head. All these motions from the head may be used in the sideways exercises, (*Fig*. 3.)

All these exercises may be further varied by carrying the arms upward as in *Fig*. 4, H and I, which can be executed only in a limited degree.

The manner in which all these positions may be combined with local walking and changing of time, we leave to the ingenuity of our readers.

To one variation, however, we call particular attention:—That the motion through the various exercises already illustrated, may be made at once instead of by measure; thus, in *Fig*. 4, the dumb bells may be carried at *one movement* from A to C and returned again, or from A to B and back again, (*Figs*. 3 and 4.)

We have been thus particular in our introduction, in order that our readers may feel themselves at home in the use of dumb bells. The description and intelligibility of the other exercises will be thereby much facilitated.

2. We introduce here the exercise of swinging the dumb bells "back and forth," making an arc of a bow shape as from G to G. The same is also to be accomplished from the point position, (*Fig*. 4, E.) In this motion of the arms above the head, when the dumb bells are swung backwards, there may be allowed a slight inclination of the body. A beautiful and useful exercise consists in holding the dumb bells at the sides of the thighs, the little finger next to the body; carry the arms sideways in such a manner as with each to cut a semi-circle in the air, the dumb bells to meet over the head, the thumbs facing one another.

3. The next exercise we introduce is called THE CLOAK. With arms outstretched in the sideways oblique position, hold the dumb bells in such a manner as that the thumbs will be opposite to each other, when the dumb bells are brought together, as at C, *Fig*. 3. Carry the arms in such a manner that the dumb bells shall describe a circle from the front, C, to the rear, as far as the build of the person exercising will permit; the letter I, *Fig*. 3, illustrates the direction in which they are carried to the rear.

4. The next exercise is a more difficult and exhausting one, styled, the SHOULDER TRIAL; see *Fig.* 4. The arms, from the hanging position, are carried forward into the horziontal position; they then separate, and each is carried slowly in a horizontal line to the sideways horizontal position, in the direction B, C, and thence back again, and thus to and fro.

This exercise serves especially for the purpose of strengthening the muscles of the breast; also to throw back the shoulder blades, and to make the chest more arched. For those whose occupation compresses the frame of the chest, the *shoulder trial* is the most appropriate means with which to counteract such tendency.

Although this exercise exerts an important influence upon the chest and its noble indwelling organs, it demands to be introduced and used with caution, especially for those who are weak and have narrow chests. A violent, jerking, backward charge of the arms, from the forward horizontal into the sideways horizontal position, is not advisable. In the beginning, it ought only to be done slowly; carrying forward in a swinging manner, can be allowed, and still later, a rapid charging back of the arms. When the arms have become accustomed to the practice of the *shoulder trial*, one may also let the lower extremities participate in some degree by lifting the body during the backward charge of the dumb bells towards *c*, so as to stand upon the ball of the foot, and thus balance one's selt upon the points of the feet and balls; but at every forward charge fall back again upon the sole of the foot. This exercise must be made in 3-3 time; thus see *Fig.* 4.

Count *One:* Arms are carried from the perpendicular position A, to the horizontal one B.

" *Two:* From the horizontal forward position B, *Fig.* 4, to the horizontal sideways position, *Fig.* 3, B.

" *Three:* Back again to the perpendicular position A, *Fig.* 4.

It is left for the pupil to decide, if he will add to this exercise local walking, in 3-3 measure with an accent on the first step.

5. The Revolving Mill Exercise, our readers will understand by examining *Fig.* 4.

4-4 time: From the hanging down position, A.
One: " " forward horizontal " B.
Two: " " upward pointing " C.
Three: In the oblique backward " D.
Four: " backward charge and arms down again.

In this manner the arm describes a circle, which becomes somewhat irregular, because the manner in which the arm is connected at the shoulder joint, does not enable it to make the backward charge in a direct line. The pupil seeks quite involuntarily to assist this, by leaning the upper part of the body over to the opposite side. The effect of this exercise upon the shoulders and chest is more useful, however, if the upper part of the body remains firm, and the arm circling backwards, is only swung as far as the anatomical build of the body will permit. The exercise may be varied by dispensing with the four movements in 4-4 time, and substituting the mill revolving, at a single sweep of the arms—first with the right arm, then with the left, and then alternately with both. It may be practiced in the circle denoted by A, H, I, C, B, the arm fronting the body in making the circle, by which the right arm goes before the body to the left, and the left moves in the opposite direction; this is practiced with alternate arms. When practiced with both arms, it is done in the most appropriate manner, with feet extended one before the other, as already designated in the *apart position*.

6. The Tunnel Circle Exercise resembles closely the preceding one, which is done in the same manner with outstretched arms, with only the difference that the circle described by the swinging dumb bell is a much smaller one. The smaller the circumference of this circle, the more difficult the exercise. It can be done with both arms, or each one alternately.

The line which is described by the exercising hand, can be a greater or smaller circular line, or a serpentine line, which widens or narrows the circle spirally.

This exercise, so varied as to describe two circles intersecting each other, in such manner as to form the figure 8, (∞) is easily understood by referring to *Fig*. 3, K.

The tunnel circle can be executed with the arms in the upward pointing position C, as well as in the horizontal B, and oblique position A. A useful variation consists in uniting the rapid tunnel circling with the *foot balancing*. The pupil takes a position upon the tips of the toes, and performs a quick sinking and rising of the heels, to follow each tunnel circling without allowing the heels to touch the floor.

7. The Arm Revolving Exercise is a motion of the arm, the object of which is to develope the mobility of the socket by means of the rolling muscles. This exercise may be undertaken from the horizontal, side-

ways position. The dumb bells are taken with the wrist grasp, *i. e.* the arms are then twisted so far as to bring the palms of the hand uppermost; this is called the *comb grasp*. Two variations of this exercise can be made, by taking the dumb bells in the *spoke grasp*, *i. e.* with the thumb uppermost; or in the *ell grasp*, with the little finger uppermost. The pupil can arrange for himself what proportion of each of these twists can be adopted best in unison with the other exercises.

B.

Elbow Exercises with Dumb Bells.

The arm and forearm are united at the elbow joint, through which is brought about the relation of the motions of the two, which in many movements are different in the two parts of the arm. The second group of dumb bell exercises are for the practice of the forearm, and are called *elbow exercises*.

1. Let us represent to ourselves the bending of the lower part of the arm, in such a manner as to cut a line, as designated by the arrow point at A, *Fig.* 5, which can be executed from the horizontal forward position, the dumb bells grasped so that the thumbs will be uppermost—the *spoke grasp*. From the horizontal position seen in figure 5, the dumb bell is carried over the points marked C, and D, to A; and the upper ball of the bell is brought near to the shoulder. It is then carried back to its original position; the upper part of the arm in this exercise remains *fixed*. This may be executed in 8-8 time, thus:

Count *One:* Bend the arm to the obtuse angle, *Fig.* 5, C.

" *Two:* Stretch it out.

Count *Three:* Bend to the right angle, D.
" *Four:* Stretch it out.
" *Five:* Bent it to an acute angle, A.
" *Six:* Stretch it out.
" *Seven:* Bend until the hand approaches to the shoulder.
" *Eight:* Stretch it out.

Alternate by *inversion.*

It is useful to vary these movements, so that the bending and stretching of the arms, alternately or simultaneously, is executed slowly, or with swinging or *jerking* motions of the arms, or with the lower part of the *arm striking out.*

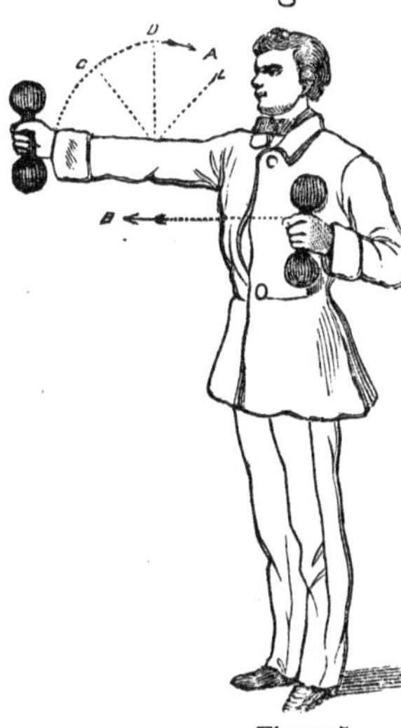

Figure 5.

2. At *Fig.* 5, the arm is in a position for the thrust. The reverse of this is the forward *thrust* or charge, when the arm is *stretched* out to its full extent, likewise in a straight line, *Fig.* 5, B. We regulate these two exercises thus: the arm is drawn in at count one; but the forward charge is in 2-2 or 3-3 time, according to how far the dumb bells are carried, whether 1-3 or 2-3 of the length to which the arm will stretch. The drawing in may be done in time divisions if desired.

Our readers will infer, from what has been previously said, how greatly this exercise may be varied.

The *twist thrust* is a variation particularly valuable. When a thrust has been made into the forward horizontal direction, spoke grasp, immediately after a short drawing back of the arm, a second thrust follows, in which the lower arm is twisted so that the thumb is thereby turned downward.

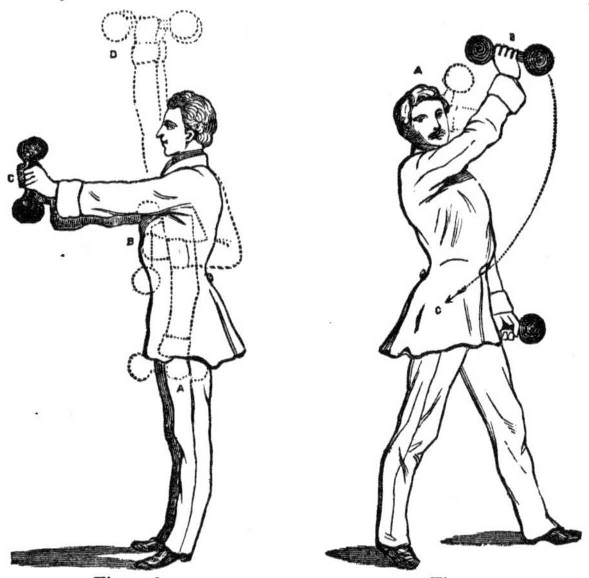

Figure 6. Figure 7.

3. An easy exercise is formed from the previous one, with the *up* and *down* charge of the dumb bells, (*Fig.* 6.) Time 4-4. From the hanging down position of the arms, A, they are drawn back, B, ready for the charge at count *one*.

Two: Arms stretched to the position seen at C.

Three: Arms drawn back for the charge, dumb bells over the shoulders, little finger uppermost.

Four: Arms charge upwards, D.

The pupil may associate with this exercise local

walking in 4-4 time, accenting count *one* with a stamp, to designate the *up* or *down* charge. It becomes still more difficult, if with the local walking in 4-4 time, be united the upward charge of the dumb bells, holding them in this position during one measure.

4. When the arms are drawn back over the shoulder, the charge is upward; when under, it is downward; when in front, it is forward.

5. We designate the exercise shown in *Fig.* 7, as the HORSEMAN'S CUT.

In this exercise, the right hand is drawn over the left shoulder, as seen in *Fig.* 7, A. From this position a vigorous blow is executed, from high to low, the arm being fully stretched at the middle of the curve B, C. It is executed with the right and left alternately. The stroke can be made upward to the shoulder, from the hips, as well as downward, commencing with the left arm.

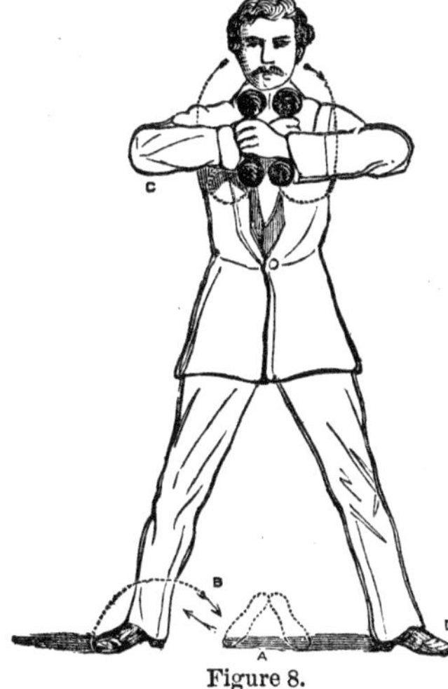

Figure 8.

6. THE FOREARM CIRCLE.

Take the bells with the spoke grasp, and bring them to the position seen in *Fig.* 8. The right arm makes a circle around the left arm, whilst the left arm makes a circle around the right arm. It may be reversed, alternated, and made more or less rapidly. The upper part of the arm is kept in the horizontal position.

7. The THRUST STRIKING EXERCISE. This is an agreeable exercise, compounded of thrusting and striking movements. It is executed in 3-3 time, thus:

Count *One*: The arms are swung from the sides, in the direction of the curve A, to the position seen in *Fig.* 9.

Two: Made to cut the curve B, C.

Three: Thrust down.

In making the upward curve, the arms should be kept perfectly straight.

C.

Hand Exercises with Dumb Bells.

There are but a limited number of these, on account of the limited action of the wrist joint. We introduce the following:

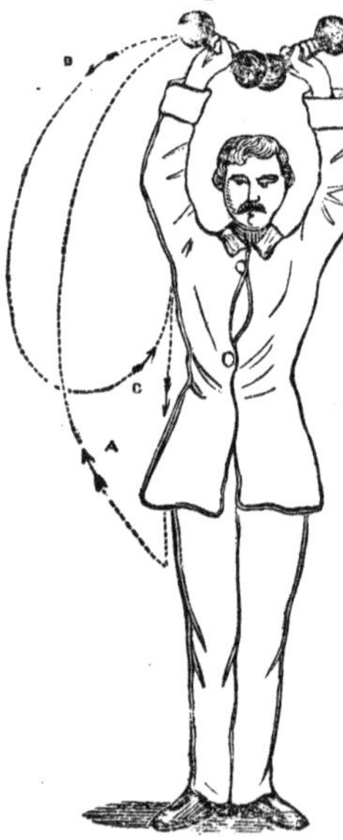

Figure 9.

1. The UPTURNING HAND EXERCISE. Take the dumb bells with the wrist grasp; now with the arms extended horizontally at the side, move the hands up and down in an easy manner, as seen in *Fig.* 3, F.

2. The HAND CIRCLING EXERCISE. Grasp the dumb bell by one ball, as seen in *Fig.* 3, E. Now describe a circle with the other ball, moving the hand around the surface of an ideal cone, the point of which lies in the wrist joint.

These exercises are very useful to those who habitually have cold hands; to those who in writing or similar labor, produce a one-sided activity of that member, or where there is a weakness in the wrist joint. They should be executed with the arms extended.

D.

Special Importance of the Dumb Bell Exercises, described in A, B, and C.

Our readers have no doubt seen, and perhaps experienced in their own persons, that the exercises already described, affect the whole muscular system, and particularly the muscles of the shoulders, arms and upper half of the trunk, in which is contained those important organs—the lungs, heart, large vessels and nerves. Upon the size of this chest cavity and the mobility of its walls, depend the perfection of respiration. Physicians ascribe those numberless diseases of the lungs and heart, including that depopulating disease, Consumption, (which carries away its millions) to a contracted chest, which lessens the space for the play of those organs contained within it. These exercises all tend to the enlargement of this cavity, and to the normal arching of its walls. The broadly arched chest of those who have had gymnastic training, forms an agreeable contrast with the weak, contracted chests of those who inherited predisposition to pulmonary affections, and who are readily recognized by their short breath, stooping forms and constant disposition to cough. As the size of the chest is increased by these exercises, so is the size of the lungs augmented, respiration perfected, and a susceptibility to those insidious diseases lessened.

A second advantage of these exercises is, that

thereby the irritability of the nerves is distributed more evenly over the body; and, as in pulmonary diseases the lungs are particularly irritable, to equalize it, is exceedingly important. If every one would make it his special care to strengthen those organs, lung diseases would become rare.

The heart is greatly improved by these exercises. With every movement its activity is accelerated, and being a muscle, like other muscles, it must increase in steadiness, size and vigor. There is a close connection between the size and power of the heart and the amount of exercise taken. Anatomists always find this organ large and firm in those who devote their lives to muscular labor, but small and flabby in those of sedentary habits.

Dumb bell exercises have an important effect on the skin. Many dangerous diseases are caused by a feeble circulation in this organ; and there exists no more effective means for securing its normal development, than vigorous muscular exercise.

To those whose organization demands special care, we advise, first those exercises described for the hands; next those for the elbows, and then those for the arms.

CHAPTER IV.

Dumb Bell Exercises with varied positions, having special reference to the Development of the Lower half of the body.

Although the arms, to some extent, participate in the exercises given in this chapter, their relation to the development of the abdominal organs, legs and feet, is the same that those given in Chapter III, sustain to the development of the chest, arms and hands. When united with a changing of the position, their scope is very great.

A.

Movements of the Leg.

1. In the previous chapter was shown, how dumb bell exercises could be combined with local walking; in this we add, that they can also be combined with walking from place to place. The exercise may be varied by walking forward two steps on *tip toe*, and alternating with two common steps. When walking on tip toe, the dumb bells should be carried in the sideways, horizontal, or oblique position; when the usual step is taken, they should be in the hanging down position.

There is one kind of walking especially adapted to unite with our dumb bell exercises, and which is practiced in 2-2 time. The pupil stands in the locked position of the feet.

Count *One:* Left foot takes one step sideways.

" *Two:* Right foot follows, and the locked position is restored. This may be varied by taking a forward step with the left foot at *one*, and following it with the right foot at *two*. When the forward step is taken with the left foot, raise the left arm to the horizontal position and let it sink down when the right foot follows; in the same manner the right arm is raised, when the right foot takes the first forward step. Finally follows the raising or thrusting out of both arms at each forward step, and the falling down or drawing back of the arms at the second step.

An exercise in which the lower extremities participate with still more energy, may be executed in this manner: First, take the forward step with a light spring or jump. Second, let the same step be a little to the left, and come down upon the point of the left foot in such a manner, that the weight will be supported by an elastic bending at the knee and foot. When the spring step is taken, swing up the dumb-bells to the sideways oblique position. When the next step is taken, which brings the support of the body on the point of the left foot, the dumb bells are to be let down again.

We introduce next an exercise more easy of execution. Feet in the locked position. Both dumb bells are taken in the manner indicated by *Fig.* 12, A. Time, 4-4 moderate. Count *one* and *two*. Raise the body upon the points of the feet, and let it down slowly upon the soles again; simultaneously with this movement, stretch out both arms to the upward pointing position, and draw them back again. Count *three*

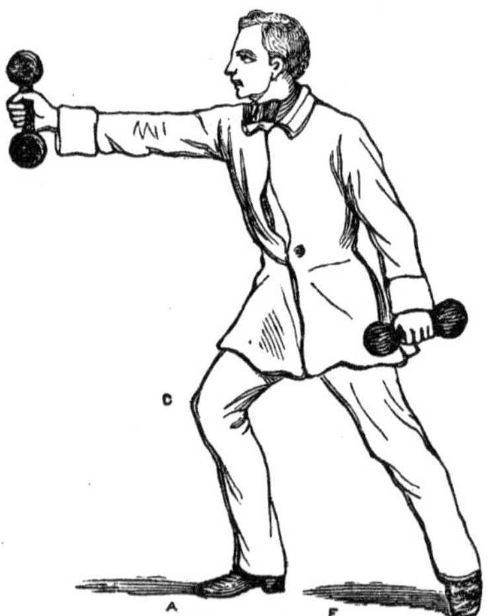

Figure 10.

and *four*; spring forward to the right or left, the arms

not in action. To this we subjoin *the triple stamp*, in which a quick movement of the feet takes place, and which may prove a remedy for cold feet. On counting *one*, three steps are taken, each one a stamp, and they follow each other rapidly: left foot down first, then right, then left. Count *two*. Back again; when right foot is down first, then left, then right. These are *sideways* steps, and the exercise may be varied by taking them forward and backward. The speed and distance of the steps may also be increased.

An exercise which is especially useful, consists in taking the forward spring step with the leg which is put forward, bent at the knee joint like *Fig*. 10, C; the upper part of the body is kept as erect as possible. Unite with this the thrusting out of the arm on the same side, as the leg which takes the forward step. The time may be regulated thus: Count *one*, *two*, to the forward step, and *three* to after step.

The different arm exercises, the *arm revolving*, *mill revolving*, *tunnel circling*, *up* and *down charging* of the dumb bells, *arm thrusting* and *arm striking*, can be united with the walking, in 3-3 or 4-4 time.

2. In this course of exercises, the free participation of the legs can take place only by their *alternate* action. In order to understand the leg exercises, our readers must refer to *Fig*. 11. The first are the *spreading out* exercises, in which the locked position of the feet is taken, and the leg moves from the hip joint—with the leg firmly stretched—either in a straight line, as much as possible in the upward pointing position, or in a semi-circle line, cone-shaped. When it moves in a straight line, the right leg is first moved sideways to a small angle, upon which the angle in the direction C,

D, E, *Fig.* 11, is gradually enlarged, perhaps to the acute angle. After each elevation of the leg, one may with a swing return it to the locked position, which movement may be regulated by time measure, if desired.

In repeating the previous exercise, may be introduced the gradual raising of the dumb bells in a similar direction. It is practiced by a continued alternation, from right to left, and left to right, the *locked* position always intervening.

A good exercise is the *leg beat*, towards the hand F, *Fig.* 11, where the dumb bells are raised to the forward horizontal position, alternately, the left and right hand; and the leg which corresponds with the outstretched arm, is swung upwards until it touches the

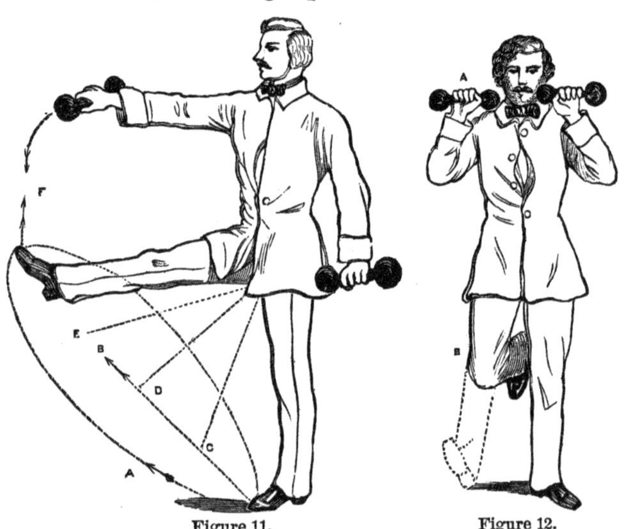

Figure 11. Figure 12.

dumb bell; this is facilitated by slightly lowering the dumb bell towards the foot.

The *bow spreading*, *Fig.* 11, A, is easily comprehended, and may be made larger or smaller, according to the size of the bow to be described. The *revolving mill* dumb bell exercise, is appropriate to be united with the *bow spreading*.

3. The exercises which result from a co-operation between the upper and lower parts of the leg, through bending at the knee joint, may be formed analogous to the elbow exercises. When the leg is lifted up, and the lower half of the leg is thereby drawn up towards the upper, this is called *lift bending* of the knees; the lower part of the leg is so far extended that the heel touches the seat; this is called the *heel touch*. Carrying the thigh up towards the abdomen, we call the *knee spring*. The *heel touch*, with both legs, simultaneously, is called the *double beat*. The *knee spring*, executed with both legs, is called the *quick double leap*.

The drawing up of the leg, and position of the foot for the push or stroke which is to follow, *Fig.* 12, C, will, in connection with the stroke, correspond with the arm-striking dumb bell exercise, which may be easily united with these leg exercises.

4. The movement which occurs when the *locked* position is changed to the *apart* position, we use, by associating with it dumb bell exercises: thus see *Fig.* 8. From the locked position, upon counting

One, the left foot moves half a step to the left.
Two, the right " " " " " right.
Three, the left " returns to its original place.
Four, the right " " " " "

At the same time that the left foot takes its step, the dumb bell in the left hand is carried up to the horizontal position of the arm: this occurs upon the *first* count.

Two, down again. *Three*, dumb bell in right hand is carried up. *Four*, down again. The movements with hands and feet are simultaneous.

This exercise may be changed by substituting the forward for the side step.

The second variation in the change of position is produced thus : whilst *one*, *two*, are counted, the change is made from the *locked* position to the *apart* position ; when *three* is counted a spring is made with both feet, simultaneously, to their first position ; the leap is to be executed as lightly as possible by coming upon the points of the feet. This transition into the apart position, and leaping back upon the points of the feet to the locked position, may be repeated in 3-3 time. The arms we make participators in such a way, that they are held in the drawn-back position, for the thrust, as at *Fig*. 6, B. When the first spring is made, both arms are thrust forward in a horizontal position ; whilst at the second step they are drawn back, and thus they continue to alternate.

A third variation of our changing positions consists in this : that the change to the apart position, and the spring back to the locked position, takes place as it is indicated by *Fig*. 8, D. The method of uniting with this the dumb bell exercises, we leave to our readers.

The changing-position exercises are of themselves very effective if executed with a spring, whilst the dumb bells remain fixed in the horizontal, oblique, or upward position.

One form of exercise we will here call attention to, where the spring, locked position and apart position alternate in such a manner that they are gradually enlarged by every change.

One: Spring from the locked position into a short apart position.

Two: Legs still more apart, by a similar movement.

Three: Legs as far apart as possible, by a similar movement.

Four: Back again to the locked position.

This exercise becomes still more effective if one returns after *each* enlarged apart position into the locked position.

5. More difficult and vigorous yet are these exercises, where the bending and stretching of the lower extremities takes place in such a manner that they have to bear the whole weight of the body.

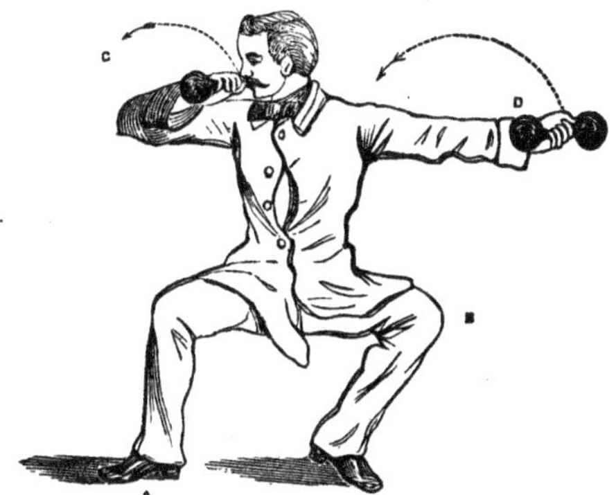

Figure 13.

This *sinking bend* of the knees is accomplished first with both legs, which are in the locked position, and by means of this bending of the knees the upper part of the body is lowered to the floor. Commence this exercise in a very moderate manner, from the attainment of a point, in which the relative position of the thigh and leg produce an obtuse angle, to one in which an acute angle is produced, and finally to one, where the thigh and leg almost touch, and the body comes close upon the ground. *(Fig. 13.)*

The *straight stretch* movement is the reverse of that which takes place in the *sinking bend*. The upper part of the body and the upper part of the leg are stretched as far distant as possible from the lower part of the leg, whilst remaining in the same direction with it. The upper part of the body must remain in an erect position.

We compose a few exercises from the *sinking bend*, and the *straight stretch*, which are particularly recommended to our dumb bell friends, and especially to the hypochondriac and to those who have a weak abdomen.

A. From the locked position, go through the three degrees of the *sinking bend*, to 3-3 time. From the squatting position reached at the third count, go through the *straight stretch* in 4-4 time, reaching the erect position at the fourth count. The arms, as in *Fig.* 13, C, are drawn back, and are in three gradations stretched until they reach the horizontal sideways position, *Fig.* 13, D. With the *straight stretch* comes the swinging bend of both arms for the drawn back position, which precedes the thrust.

B. The sinking bend position, through the three degrees, down to the squatting position, takes place when *one* is counted. *Two*, *three* and *four* indicate successively the three degrees which follow the straight stretch; the third count finds the pupil erect. The accompanying dumb bell exercise for this is the same as in A, but in a reversed order.

C. Each *sinking bend* of greater or lesser angle is followed each time by a stretch position. In 6-6 time, the three degrees in sinking bend may take place respectively upon *one*, *three* and *five*. Two, four and six indicate three degrees of the straight stretch; this exercise may be repeatedly performed. From what has already been written, our readers will be able to devise the appropriate dumb bell exercises to accompany these exercises of the leg and body.

D. The *sinking bend* may also, in 6-6 time, alternate in such a manner with the *straight stretch*, that when *one* is counted, the squatting position of the sinking bend is taken; while, when two, four and six are counted, the rising up, in degrees of the *straight stretch* is accomplished.

E. From the *apart position*, the sinking bend and straight stretch involve a more vigorous exercise, and one which is at the same time more effective for the lower limbs.

F. The *sinking bend*, executed in such a way that the whole weight of the body rests more especially upon one leg, is a more difficult exercise, and should only be undertaken after both legs have been for some time subject to practice. To accomplish this, one leg takes the forward step position, *Fig.* 13, A, and supports the other, B, when the latter, in a similar manner and connection as in the sinking bend exercise executed with both legs, assumes the principal labor; right and left are to be practiced, and to be united with dumb bell exercises as indicated by *Fig.* 13.

G. Finally, we recommend to our readers an exercise of more easy execution, in the following form: Position—the body balanced upon the points of the feet; exercise: the *sinking bend;* this may be alternated with the sole of the feet on the floor. Two steps can be taken forward, and two back again; or two can be taken sideways, right and left to 4-4 time. Also in 2-2 or 3-3 time, the sinking bend and straight stretch exercises may be connected with the dumb bell exercise from the drawn back position, whence may be executed the horizontal sinking down or thrusting out movements.

All the exercises which have been executed thus far, (especially those under 5,) provoke a vigorous and uniform action of the muscles of the legs. They acquire their physiological importance, from their being the means of exciting to action the functions of the abdomen, and especially the process of digestion.

6. As our readers are already acquainted with the *stepping forward* position, the *sally*, (*Fig*. 10,) we now give an exercise which resembles the *thrust strike*, B, *Fig*. 7, and which is called the *thrust throw*, (*Fig*. 14.) From the *locked position*, when *one* is counted, the dumb bells are carried back as far as designated by *Fig*. 14, D. *Two!* Swung forward in the direction pointed by the arrow at B, and are brought into a position by the sides of the chest, where they will be ready for the next movement. *Three!* The dumb bells are thrust forward horizontally as at C. Simultaneous with the *thrust throw* takes place the stepping out and bending movement of alternate legs. This exercise is repeated in the following manner: *One!* The dumb bells are carried with outstretched arms in the direction A; backward again, simultaneously with the return of the foot and leg which had taken the forward step to the locked position. The thrust throw is continued in this manner in 3-3 time.

7. *Fig*. 14 explains the BOXING EXERCISE. When *one* is counted, take the position seen at C,

Fig. 14. *Two!* The *thrust-out* takes place precisely as in *Fig*. 14, accompanied with stepping out.

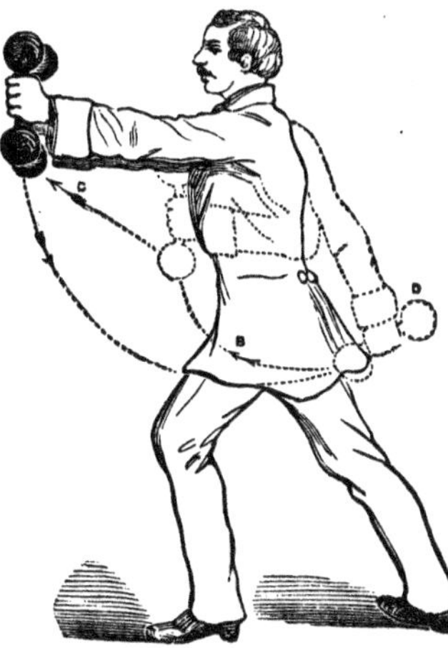

Figure 14.

8. A third exercise upon *Fig*. 14, is a beautiful one. The dumb bells are held in a forward horizontal position, (*Fig*. 14, C) ; the feet in the locked position. Count *One:*— With the left foot step forward to the fall out position, simultaneously both arms are swung backwards, as in the *shoulder trial*, (*Fig*. 4, A.) Count *Two:* The foot returns to the locked position, the dumb bells being at the same time carried forward to the horizontal position.

9. An entertaining and effective exercise is catching the dumb bell. The position for this is illustrated in *Fig*. 10, K. The dumb bell is held with the wrist grasp so that the wrist joint is highest; let it fall, but catch it again with a sudden grasp. It may be permitted to fall lower and lower, as one becomes practiced in the exercise. It may also be practiced with the fall-out step to the left.

10. As a very useful, though fatiguing exercise, we will introduce the GRASS HOPPER LEAP. The *squatting position*, (*Fig*. 13, B,) is taken; the knees are kept firmly together, and one hops with both legs. With the first leap, the dumb bells are swung back, (*Fig*. 14, A,) but at the second leap, they are carried to the upward position.

B.

Body Movements.

In the dumb bell exercises which have been described thus far, the limbs have been especially called into activity, and they embody to a considerable degree the body movements, especially with the arms. Physiological considerations render it important that a thorough exercise of the muscles of the back be provided for, and for this purpose we describe some amusing exercises.

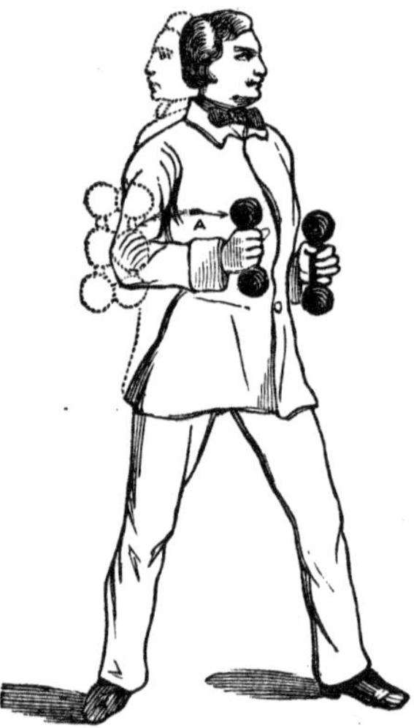

Figure 15.

1. The TWIST SWING is a simple exercise, and is executed from the apart position. The dumb bells are held as seen in *Fig.* 15, hands close to each other; they are carried in a swinging manner, first to the right, then to the left, accompanied by a twisting of the whole body. After a short time, the dumb bells can be held at a greater distance from the body, which will make the trunk-twisting more vigorous.

2. The BOW SWINGING, (*Fig.* 16.) must also be executed from the apart position, and with it the upper part of the body must be bent forward; the arms hang down, the thumbs towards each other, and the dumb bells are swung in a large semi-circle to the right and to the left, as seen in *Fig.* 16. The whole body follows the motion of the dumb bells, by turning first to one side and then to the other. The feet twist themselves at the same time in

this manner: with the bow spring to the left, the point of the left foot turns to the left; and with the bow spring to the right, the point of the right foot turns to the right. The curve swept by the dumb bells extends from near the floor as high as the head.

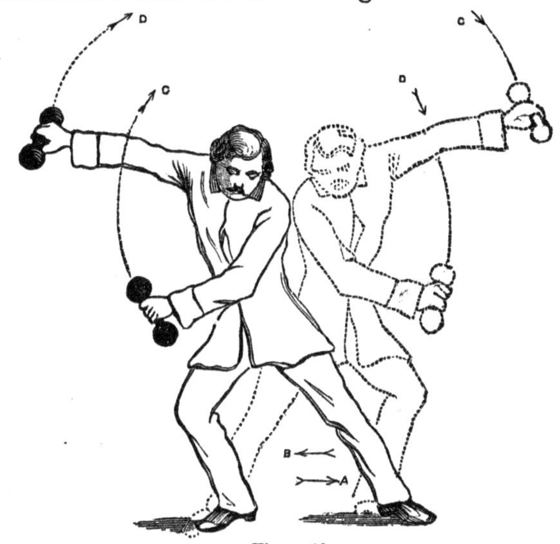

Figure 16.

3. The BOW MILL EXERCISE. The apart position is taken, from which the dumb bells are made to describe a circle, the circumference of which shall be as near as possible to the floor, and as high up on the right as possible, and thus is followed by another circle of the same description to the left.

4. The TRANSFER OF DUMB BELLS. This is an entertaining and effective exercise, which is made plain by a study of *Fig*. 17. The far-apart position is taken; the dumb bells are removed from left to right, and right to left, as far as possible.

Taking up and *putting down* the dumb bells: this

may appropriately follow the preceding exercise, and may be used at any time when in the course of his exercises the pupil wishes to put his dumb bells down. *One*, by a spring changes his position from the locked to the apart position, and with a bending movement of the body at the same moment, places the dumb bells

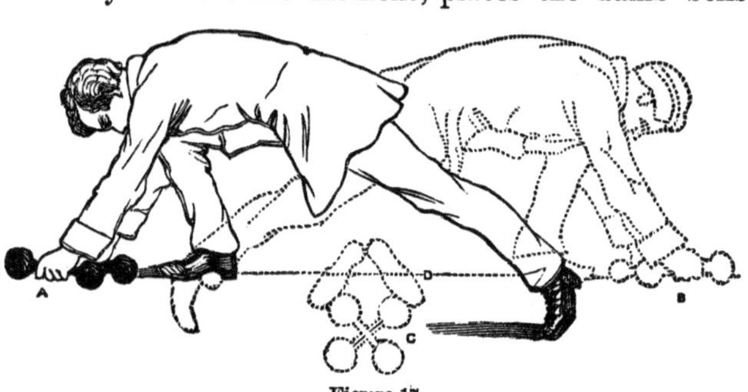

Figure 17.

crossways before him, (*Fig.* 17 C.) He returns at once with a spring into the locked position, D, body erect. *Taking up* the dumb bells, occurs in a similar manner, by a rapid change from the apart to the locked position.

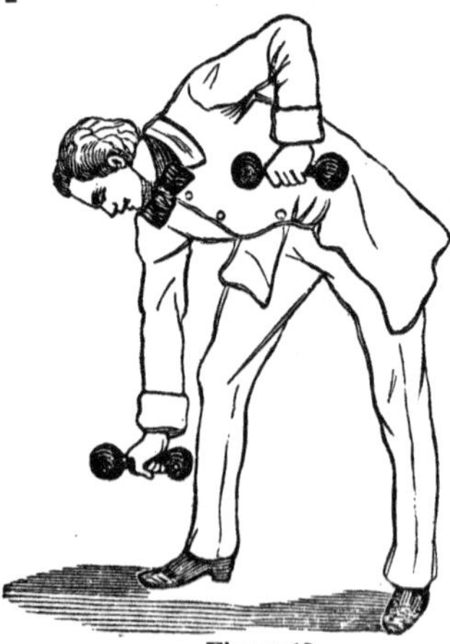
Figure 18.

6. The STAMPING EXERCISE, (*Fig.* 18,) is executed from the apart position, with the body bent forward; the arms are drawn back and thrust forward alternately, as illustrated in *Fig.* 18.

7. The WOOD SAWYER is an exercise of an amusing nature. From the lock position (with the dumb

bells held in the upward pointing position) spring to the apart position, and bring the dumb bells down to a point between the legs. The dumb bells are then swung up again and at the same time the apart position is resumed. Time 2-2. (*Fig.* 19.)

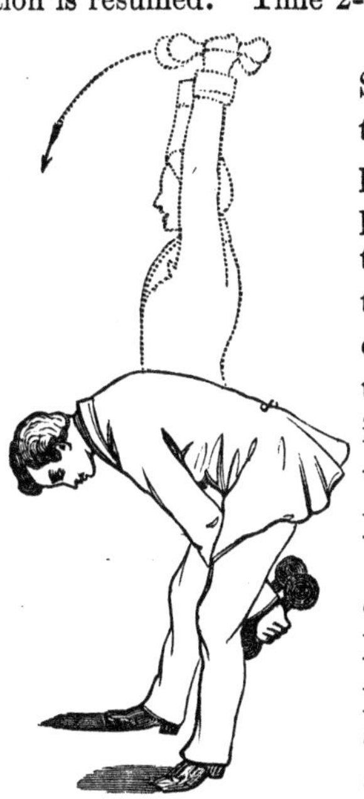

Figure 19.

8. The Up and Down Spring Exercise is similar to the preceding one. The pupil springs into the apart position, whilst also assuming the squatting position; and the dumb bells are laid at either side of the feet. From this position he springs up into the erect ones, carrying up the dumb bells to the position indicated in *Fig.* 19.

We close this series of exercises with the Rocking Leap, (*Fig.* 20.) to accomplish which one must have already acquired considerable agility. The position is plainly indicated in the cut. The left foot is forward at point C; the dumb bells are held in the horizontal forward position; the two arcs of a circle are described in succession, first by the left foot from C to A, followed almost simultaneously by the right foot to B; the right foot then becomes the forward one. Whilst this change of position is being accomplished, the dumb bells are drawn in as indicated by the dotted line, and thrust out again as soon as the change is accomplished. One performs this movement from right to left, and from left to right. It is a beautiful exercise.

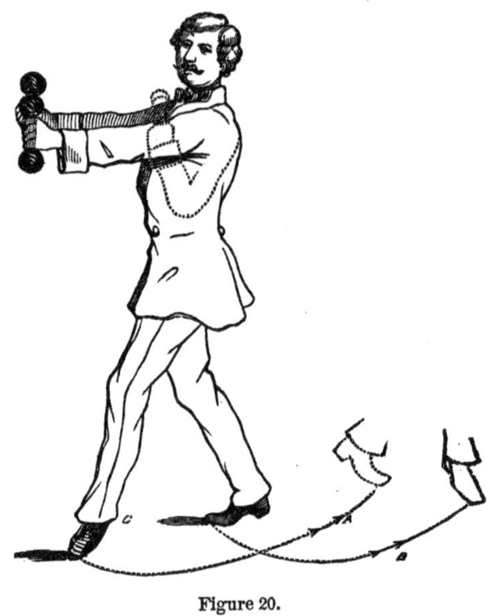

Figure 20.

C.

Special Importance of these Dumb Bell Exercises.

Laxity of the hip, abdomen and back, is a more frequent cause of diseases affecting the liver, stomach and bowels, and of hysteria and hypochondria, than is usually supposed. To preserve these organs in health, and to cure them when diseased, these muscles must be thoroughly invigorated. This is most effectually accomplished by the exercises given in this chapter. They are highly recommended by physicians for the removal of constipation, piles, dyspepsia, flatulency, intestinal rheumatism, &c. For the sedentary they are especially valuable, as they are frequent subjects of these diseases.

CHAPTER V.

Restrictions in the use of Dumb Bells, to be observed by Invalids.

Invalids should calculate closely the amount of exercise they can bear. They should also be careful in selecting what is adapted to their wants. It will be well for them to consult their family physician on this point. Physicians of late years have not only given attention to gymnastics as a means of preserving health, but they also prescribe them for relieving and curing many diseases. To them it will not be difficult to designate those which must be avoided, and such as will answer the requirements of the patient.

Our dumb bell exercises have particular reference to pulmonary and abdominal diseases. Of the former Prof. RICHTER observes, that "Gymnastics may prove a valuable remedy; or, they may do great injury." Where there exists tubercles in the lungs, expansion of the thorax is important; where asthmatic disease exists, in which the lungs tend to enlarge beyond their normal size, contraction is desirable. To both these conditions, gymnastic exercises are applicable.

Dumb bell arm exercises, with deep inhalations for enlarging the upper part of the chest, can be recommended where tubercles have begun to form. Where the adhesive state has been reached, great caution is necessary, in order to avoid laceration or hemorrhage. They should not be continued so as to produce palpitation of the heart, or congestion of the lungs. Where tubercles are far advanced, no exercises which call into action the muscles of the thorax should be used; but those which affect the lower part of the arm, or at most the bending and stretching exercise for the upper part of the arm, all these must be executed very slowly. The following succession may be observed:

1. The HAND EXERCISES, in a position that will not produce too much exertion—the *oblique downward* position.

2. The following from among the ELBOW EXERCISES:

A. The bending and stretching of the lower part of the arms: first, in the hanging down position; then in the oblique; and lastly in the horizontal position.

B. The *lower arm circling*, (Chapter III, B, B,) first with hanging down, and then with raised elbows.

C. The *up* and *down changing* of the dumb bells, (Chapter III, B, 3.)

3. The following from among the ARM EXERCISES:

A. Carrying the dumb bells up to the oblique, and then to the horizontal sideways position.

B. The *bow swing* exercise, from the hanging down position.

C. The *cloak* exercise.

D. The *mill revolving*.

E. The *tunnel circle*.

These exercises must be brought into use gradually, as the patient is able to bear them; and difficult ones, affecting the chest, must not be introduced until these have produced considerable relief. For tuberculated lungs, the chief benefit is afforded by such training as shall increase the inhalation.

Dumb bell exercises must not be practiced by persons having diseases of the heart, or blood vessels; and all exercises which have a heating tendency, should be avoided by those suffering with diseases of the blood. In affections of the brain and spine, such of those movements, as would be prescribed by a judicious physician, will prove valuable.

The prejudice against gymnastics for those who have rupture, is not well founded. As a laxity of the abdominal muscles often predisposes to this disease, so exercises which invigorate these muscles, tend to contract the abdominal ring, and even to close it. Although exercising without the advice of a physician is not recommended in these cases, yet a slow execution of those movements which twist and bend the body, together with those which call into action the muscles of the thigh and abdomen, may generally be indulged.

CHAPTER VI.

Series of Dumb Bell Exercises for Ordinary, Every Day Use.

In selecting a group of dumb bell exercises which shall be adapted to meet the demands of daily life, it is necessary to obtain such a combination of series as shall tend to develop all the muscles of the system. By this it will be understood, that such a selection is to be avoided as would tend only to develop isolated groups of muscles. Adults, especially, will need to arrange their exercises, so that action and development may take place with the muscles connected with the abdominal and respiratory organs.

Those who have taken pains to acquaint themselves practically with our directions and disciplines of the dumb bell exercises, will find it easy to arrange the exercises according to their requirements. However, we will take occasion to arrange a few series, in order to indicate what are the right combinations for reaching, through their use, a full, harmonic, physical development.

A.

A Lesson for Beginners.

1. Raise the dumb bells from the *hanging down* to the *oblique sideways* position and back again, four to six times.

2. The same movement, but carried up as far as the *horizontal sideways* position, four to six times.

3. The exercise named *the cloak;* when the dumb bells are being swung back, rise on the toes, six to eight times.

4. Draw up the dumb bells as far as the arm-pit, and then carry them downwards to the *hanging down* position. As they are drawn *up*, the legs take the *sinking bend* position; and as the dumb bells are brought *down*, the exerciser takes the *straight stretch* position. Eight to ten times.

5. From the position designated in *Fig.* 18, carry the dumb bells through the *bow swinging* exercise, (*Fig.* 18, D, B.) This is to be done six or eight times, and connected with the straightening of the upper part of the body, and also with putting down the dumb bells as described in Chapter IV, B, 5.

6. In 3-3 time: From the *hanging down* position, raise the dumb bells to the *horizontal sideways* position, as in *Fig.* 3. Carry them to the *horizontal forward* position, (*Fig.* 4,) and return them to the *hanging down* position. Six or eight times.

7. Time, 4-4. From the *locked* position with the arms as in *Fig.* 12, move into the *apart* position, and accompany the movement with carrying the dumb bells in the *horizontal sideways* direction. Return to the

locked position, drawing back the dumb bells, from four to six times. Repeat this exercise in 3-3 time, with a spring into the *locked* position, four to six times.

8. *Sinking bend* of the leg, as described in Chapter IV, A, 5, A. At the same time the arms are raised to the *horizontal sideways* position, (Chapter III, A, 1.) Three to four times.

N. B.—Finish this series of exercise by commencing with number *eight*, and returning to number *one*, executing each exercise *once* only.

B.

A Lesson for those who are Somewhat Advanced.

1. Charging of the dumb bells *up* and *down*, Chapter III, B, 3. Eight to ten times.

2. The *thrust strike;* in such a manner that the spring into the *apart* position occurs with the swinging up of the dumb bells; and the spring into the *locked* position occurs with the downward swing of the dumb bells. Four to six times.

3. *Each arm* and *both arms*, in alternation, are bent to the various angles, illustrated in *Fig.* 5, C, D, E. Three or four times.

4. *Forward step;* walk with falling out position, 3-3 time, Chapter IV, A, 1, and arm thrusting, six times to the left and six times to the right.

5. *Double leap;* Chapter A, 3, united with stretching out the arms in the *oblique sideways* position. Four to six times.

6. The *transfer* of dumb bells, (*Fig.* 17.) Ten to twelve times.

7. *Leg beat*, towards the hand, (*Fig.* 11, F.) Six times to the left and six times to the right.

8. *Thrust throw*, with sally, (*Fig.* 14.) Six to eight times.

N. B.—Same as the previous N. B.

C.

A Lesson for Pupils still more Advanced.

1. *Shoulder trial*, united with the sally: *falling out* position, Chapter IV, A, 8. Eight to ten times.

2. *Sinking bend;* (*Fig.* 13;) more especially upon one leg, united with the *thrusting out* of the dumb bells. Three to four times.

3. *Wood Sawyer*. Eight to ten times.

4. *Knee spring*, with horizontal position of the arms. Four to six times.

5. *Bow mill*, (*Fig.* 16, 5.) Three times from left to right and three times from right to left.

6. The last exercise, Chapter IV, A, 4. Transition into the *apart* position, enlarging it; springing back each time into the *locked* position, united with lifting up and down the dumb bells with outstretched arms. Four to six times.

7. *Lower arm circling* with raised elbows, (*Fig.* 8,) swinging six times from forward to backward and six times the other way.

8. *Rocking leap;* with arm thrusting to left and right. Six to eight times.

N. B.—As before.

Every one is enabled, through the simple indications given in Chapter III and IV of our dumb bell instructor, to select that which is best adapted to his wants and that which he enjoys most. With his own ingenuity he can arrange such a series of exercises as will prove invigorating.

THE

PANGYMNASTIKON;

OR,

All Gymnastic Exercises brought within the Compass of a Single Piece of Apparatus, as the Simplest Means for the Complete Development of Muscular Strength and Endurance,

BY

D. G. M. SCHREBER, M. D.,

Director of the Medical Gymnastic Institution at Leipsic.

Illustrated with 107 Wood Cuts.

TRANSLATED FROM THE GERMAN BY DIO LEWIS, M. D.

Note by the Translator.—It is hardly fair to call this a translation, so much has it been condensed. But I am confident the form in which it is presented will prove more acceptable to the American mind, than would a faithful, full translation of the elaborate original. It should be mentioned that not only have considerable chapters been omitted, but some additions have been made; all of which is most respectfully submitted.

FORTHCOMING

MOVEMENT CURE WORKS.

Chronic maladies are found in nearly every American family. Weak spines, lungs and stomachs are well-nigh universal. Oceans of drugs have not improved us. A desire for restoration and a conviction of its possibility are general.

No thoughtful mind can study the great Swede without the undoubting faith that in his philosophy is found the hope of invalidism. The *loss of balance in muscle and in the circulation of the fluids, which is the essential condition of all chronic disease, is, with the most complete directness and success, overcome by the Swedish Movement Cure.*

Within three years I shall publish *Five Works* devoted to the Movement Cure Treatment of Chronic Maladies :—

"AFFECTIONS OF THE ORGANS OF THE CHEST, WITH THEIR TREATMENT BY THE MOVEMENT CURE."

"AFFECTIONS OF THE ORGANS OF THE ABDOMEN, WITH THEIR TREATMENT BY THE MOVEMENT CURE."

"SPINAL CURVATURES AND OTHER DEFORMITIES, WITH THEIR TREATMENT BY THE MOVEMENT CURE."

"AFFECTIONS OF THE SEXUAL SYSTEM, WITH THEIR TREATMENT BY THE MOVEMENT CURE."

"AFFECTIONS OF THE NERVOUS SYSTEM, WITH THEIR TREATMENT BY THE MOVEMENT CURE."

The first of these works will be issued before the close of the present year.

Each of the forthcoming books will contain from two to three hundred cuts. The explanations and directions will be made so simple, and the illustrative cuts so numerous and complete, that any home may become a Movement Cure for the restoration of its invalids.

My heart is filled with the hope that through these works, thousands who have vainly sought relief in medicines and journeyings, may escape their sufferings, and again enjoy the many blessings of our earthly life.

Most Respectfully,

DIO LEWIS, M. D.

INTRODUCTION.

We welcome German gymnastics as an earnest of a revival of the ancient, German, national spirit. During the long centuries of the dark ages, the Germanic soul struggled with ignorance and superstition; culminating at length in the "Thirty Year's War," during which, four-fifths of the German people were destroyed, and numberless towns utterly annihilated. At last, the worst of all possible results befel the German nation, in the suffocation of its national life. Until the year 1618, the German national spirit still existed, though restrained in its manifestations. There was a noble consciousness of physical and spiritual strength. This consciousness had been preserved through the military habits of the people.

Arms were kept in every house. Target shooting was universal. Women and children became comrades in arms. Physical vigor was an object of general emulation. Every house in town and country had its bath-room; organized and incorporated bodies superintended the bath. They were known as the "Society of Bathers." Numberless sports were introduced, and received the patronage of the government. The present English habits are to some extent a reflection of the German life during the period of which we speak. Of all these beautiful blossoms of the German national life, none survived that dreadful war. During a long reign of terror, this noble people was overwhelmed by hordes of foreign tyrants, who reduced the German nation to a shrivelled, timid, narrow-minded people, smirking and bowing down to foreigners. A long, long time elapsed ere a few small flames began to kindle in the mass of smouldering ruins, in whose depths the national spirit of olden time had yet continued to glimmer and glow. Two centuries passed, before the regeneration of the German national life could commence. All praise to God, the present generation has crossed the threshold of the new era. The new creation received its noblest impulse through the priceless labors of Gutsmuths, Jahn, Eiselen, Spiess and their fellow workers, who inaugurated the present gymnastic revolution.

Gymnastics are therefore not a mere passing thing of fashion, but a renovated, enobled instinct or germ, from the old, yet vigorous root of the ancient German national life.

Man may indulge lofty conceptions and aspirations, but without physical vigor he must ever prove a very imperfect being—a tree which bears forced blossoms and dwarfed fruit. What is true of the individual is true of a nation.

What the primary school has accomplished for the intellectual life of the nation, the gymnasium is achieving for its physical life. The primitive and aimless field sports no longer suffice. The intellectual life of the nation having reached a higher plane, system and science are demanded for its physical development. Besides, the demands made by a higher mental culture are so manifold and absorbing, as not to allow sufficient time for the primitive exercises which belong to field-sports.

The Pangymnastikon.

In this work, it is my purpose to present the claims and elaborate the uses of the *Pangymnastikon*, so called because it possesses the advantages of all other gymnastic apparatus. I would not underrate the value of other apparatus and modes of exercise. Holding the position of president of one of the oldest and most advanced gymnastic clubs in Germany, and deeply impressed with the importance of constant variety and change in apparatus and exercises, I offer the Pangymnastikon, not as a full response to the public demand, but as the most complete "multum in parvo" in the gymnastic field, and as most admirably adapted to the wants of those who cannot avail themselves of the advantages of a gymnastic institution. To all such it is a God-send.

Special Claims of the Pangymnastikon.

It is comparatively easy to devise gymnastic exercises which shall interest a social class, enlivened by music. But what shall those do, who, finding it inconvenient or disagreeable to visit the gymnasium, would cultivate muscle and vigor at home? In the absence of social stimulus and music, the exercises themselves must possess peculiar fascination. If, in addition, they bring every part of the body into varied action, giving the left arm, shoulder—the entire left half of the body as much and as varied exercise as the right, we should have the model home gymnastics.

The Pangymnastikon meets these indications more

successfully than any other apparatus yet devised. While the first exercises of the first series are simple enough for children, the last exercises of the last series are beyond the reach of all except those who have a favorable composition, and are very much in earnest. For clergymen, ladies and many others, who would carry on the work at home, this invention is the most complete means imaginable.

Description of the Pangymnastikon.

Two large hand rings suspended from the ceiling by ropes, which, running through padded hooks, are carried to the walls. Two other ropes extend from the walls directly to the hand rings. A strap with a stirrup is placed in either hand ring. By a simple arrangement on the wall, the hand-rings are drawn as high as the performer can reach, or let down within a foot of the floor; or at any altitude they can be drawn apart to any distance. The distance between the stirrups and rings can be likewise varied. The usefulness of the Pangymnastikon depends upon the facility with which these changes can be made. The rings must be raised, let down, drawn apart, the stirrup straps changed, or removed altogether from the rings, each and all with a single motion of the hand, and in a moment. There are various simple mechanical contrivances by which these multifarious changes can be made. An ingenious mechanic can scarcely be at fault. I will suggest that in splicing the ropes into the rings, the splice should be long and drawn close; else giving way, an unpleasant surprise may occur. The ropes should run through strong, padded hooks at the ceiling, which are fastened on the upper side of the timber with thick nuts. The fastenings on the wall must be made secure.

The ropes with which the rings are separated, should be armed with wrought-iron snap-hooks, which can be caught into wrought-iron rings, which have been firmly lashed into the suspension rope, at the point where it connects with the hand ring. The stirrup straps must be of very strong white leather, with edges so rounded that the pants will not be worn. In shortening the straps, a buckle should not be used, for, in removing the straps from the hand rings, much time would thereby be lost; nor should a simple hook be employed, as the leather is liable to give way, and the hook to slip out. A brass H, with one side sewed into the end of the strap doubled, and the other slipped through slits in the body of the strap, is a perfect thing. With this simple contrivance, the strap can be altered or taken out altogether in a second, and can never give way. The stirrups should be very strong, with serrated bottoms, and fastened into the ends of the straps with strong sewing and copper rivets.

The Pangymnastikon cannot be put up in an ordinary gymnasium; the ceiling is too high. The best height for the ceiling hooks is twelve feet; a ceiling as low as eight feet will do. The apparatus can be used, however, in a gymnasium, or in an open yard, by the erection of a simple frame work. If suspended in an ordinary gymnasium, from a ceiling eighteen or twenty feet high, a large number of the most valuable exercises cannot be performed advantageously.*

* If the mechanic has difficulty in understanding the processes of manufacturing the article, he may obtain full explanations by addressing Dr. Dio Lewis, Box 12, Boston, Mass., whose manufacturer will send full particulars. Persons who would prefer to obtain the Pangymnastikon at the factory in Boston, can address Dr. Lewis, who has them so made that they will not give out at any point, even after being used for years in the roughest manner and by the heaviest men. Made thus, handsomely finished, and boxed ready for shipment, the cost is $10, which is very cheap. Directions for putting it up in any room, even a parlor, without marring the ceiling or wall, will be sent with the apparatus. It can be easily removed out of the way in a moment when not wanted. **Four large sheets of cuts will be sent with it. The height of ceiling and width of room must be sent to us.**

Uses and Value of the Pangymnastikon.

Upon a close examination of the Pangymnastic exercises, the conviction will be forced upon all, that by no other means can such a variety of valuable exercises be reached.

A vain boasting over muscular strength is vulgar. I regard with disfavor the cultivation of mere strength, without a noble carriage, freedom, security, agility and grace. Still less do I approve of a mere display of feats. But what thoughtful person can reflect upon the objects of human life, without seeing that not only is the highest development of the muscular system a great advantage to those who follow mechanical occupations, but of vital importance likewise to those who fill the ranks of intellectual life, and who require as a condition of success, good health and strong vitality. Only a *whole* man is capacitated to perform in the best manner the tasks of life. Is it not an aim worthy our highest efforts to develope our whole being to its fullest capacity? To carry forward to full fruition those germs, which, like the slumbering buds of a plant, exist within us, awaiting the period of their development and ripening. That which man is in himself, that which he possesses in his own person—his intellectual and physical capabilities, constitute his only permanent, reliable capital! If then a method is opened for the development of his physical strength, not at the cost, but to the advantage of his intellectual powers, would he not prove himself a simpleton if he refused to follow such a path?

The anatomist, in examining the exercises here introduced, will not fail to discover that each and every set of muscles has received studied attention, while at the same time the general development of *the* MAN has been kept in view.

This universal development is especially provided for in the Pangymnastikon by the union of the stirrups with the rings, from which results an infinite combination and variety of exercises. The main value of the Pangymnastikon rests upon this union of the stirrups with the rings. I believe the gymnasium receives in this apparatus a larger circumference than is offered by all other gymnastic utensils combined.

The muscles of the lower part of the body, and the nape of the neck, are more thoroughly trained than by any other means. The extensor muscles of the fingers, hands, arms and legs, which are never brought into vigorous play with other gymnastic apparatus, enjoy, in the use of this apparatus, full play. The rotatory and diagonal movements of the muscles, which are particularly effective in the production of symmetry, figure prominently.

Pangymnastic exercises derive great advantage from the fact that the points of support as well as the points of grasp are moveable, whilst ordinarily these points are fixed. The advantage of the Pangymnastikon is, that these points are fixed through a varied action of the muscles. This compels an almost infinite multiplication of the direction and manner of muscular exertion.

The Pangymnastikon, as I am convinced by a wide experience, possesses strong attractions to lovers of gymnastic exercises, on account of this great variety, and the graduated difficulties to be overcome. It will everywhere prove a source of unlimited interest in private houses.

Nothing could be more admirably adapted to ships,

where invigorating exercises are greatly needed to preserve health and to prevent sea sickness.

The Pangymnastikon is therefore to become the means of an unlimited generalization of the gymnasium.

The pupil must observe the gradual method of advancing. Beginning with the most simple, and at last reaching the most difficult. He must proceed from exercise to exercise, from degree to degree, from series to series.

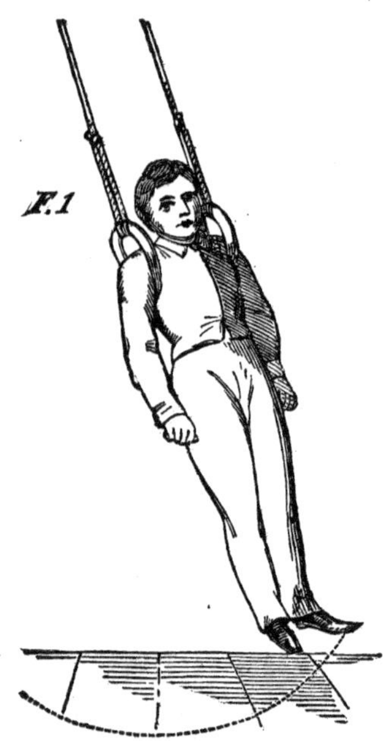

FIRST SERIES.

***Fig.* 1.** SHOULDER SWING, *forward and backward, four, six, or eight times.*

Rings at the height of the head. The swing motion

is obtained by springing from the floor, and a continued effort of the legs.

Fig. 2. ELBOW SWING, *forward and backward*, *four*, *six*, *or eight times*.

Rings high enough for the body to hang straight, the body being supported by the elbows. Swing the same as in *Fig.* 1.

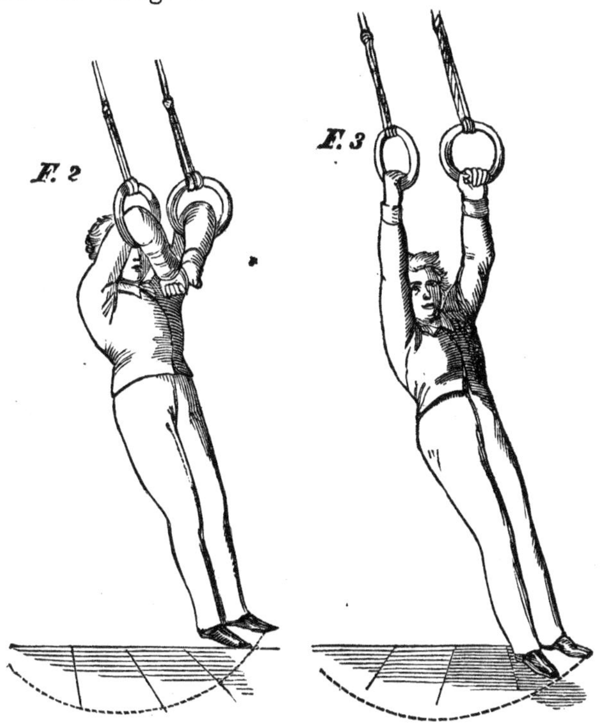

Fig. 3. HAND SWING, *forward and backward*, *four*, *eight*, *or twelve times*.

Rings so high that the feet will not touch in swinging; with the arms straight.

Fig. 4. HAND SWING SIDEWISE, *four, eight, or twelve times.*

Rings same as in the last. The swinging which is sidewise, is carried on by efforts of the legs and arms. This exercise operates happily by enlarging the chest.

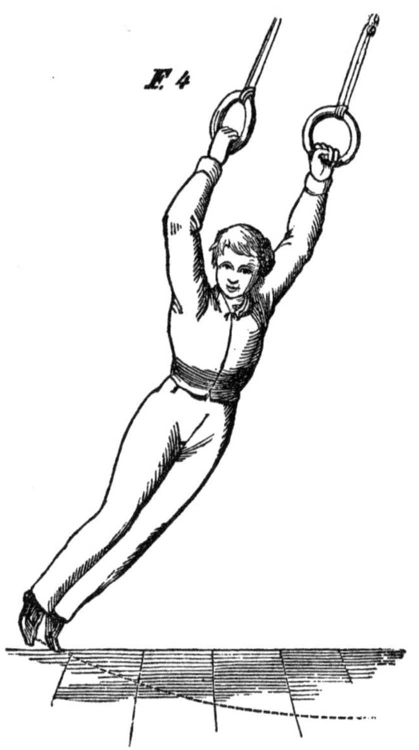

Fig. 5. STANDING INCLINATION, *forward and backward, two, four, or eight times.*

Rings as high as the chest. Seize the rings as shown in the cut. The feet remain at one place, simply turning on the toes as the person falls forward, and on the heels as he falls backward. In falling forward it is well, for beginners especially, to keep the arms in the attitude seen in the cut. The legs must not be bent.

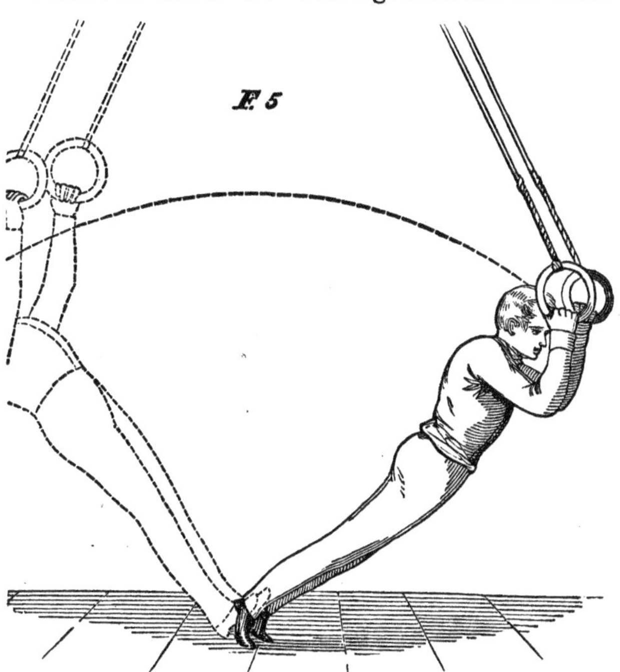

Fig. 6. STANDING INCLINATION SIDEWISE, *two, four, or eight times.*

Rings and grasp the same as in the last. The inclination of the body is exactly to the right and left alternately. The arms remain in the position shown. The body remains inflexible.

Fig. 7. TUNNEL CIRCLING, *with Shoulder Support, four, eight, or twelve times.*

Rings a hand's breadth below the height of the shoulder. Arms put through the rings; feet do not leave their position. The exercise consists in circling the body around, from left to right and from right to left, the same number of times each way. From all parts of the circle, the body faces in the same direction. The body must not be allowed to bend in the least.

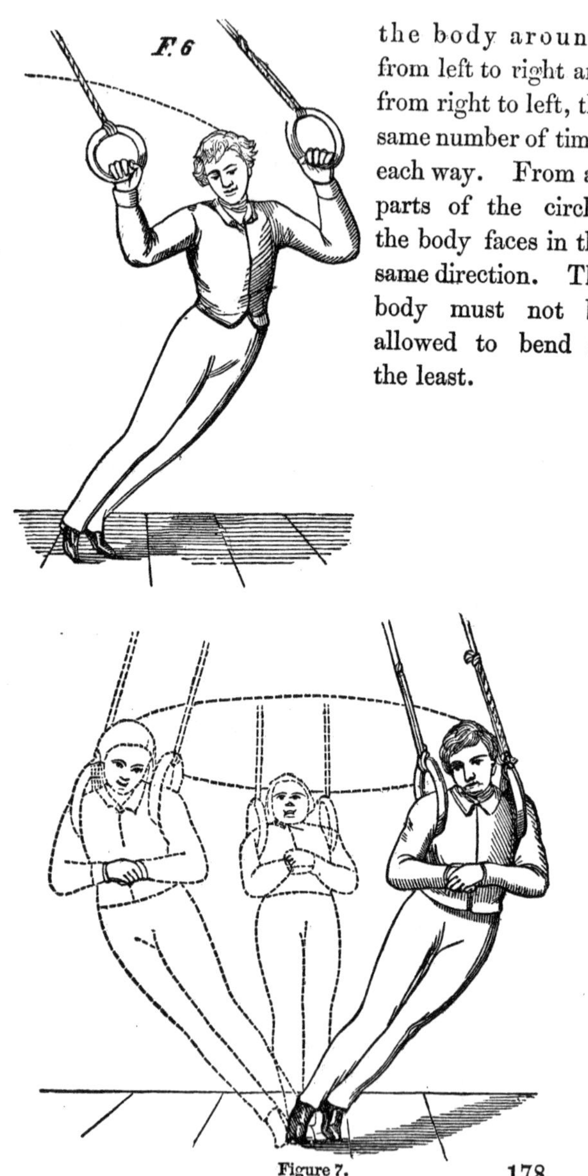

Figure 7.

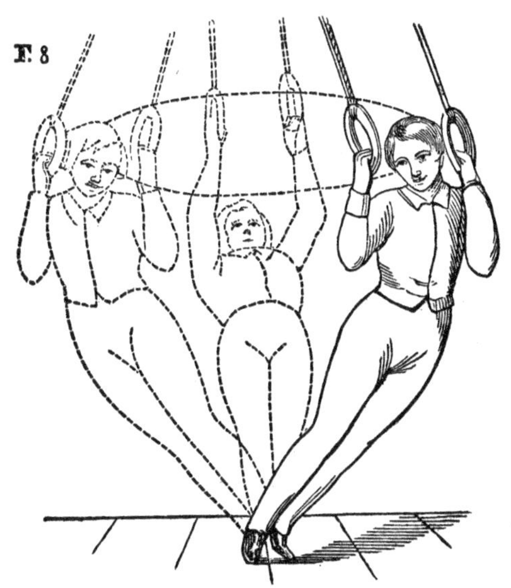

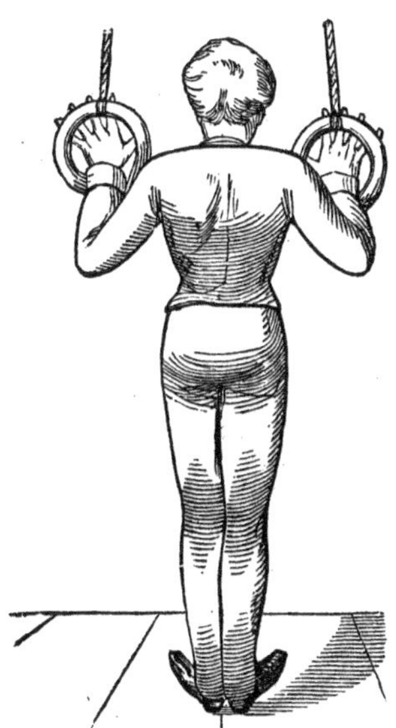

Figure 9.

Fig. 8. TUNNEL CIRCLING *with Hand Grasp, two, four, or six times.*

Rings at the height of the shoulder. The rings being taken in the hands, the circle is larger and the muscular exertion greater. The lower the rings are placed, the greater will be the muscular exertion. The body must not be allowed to turn upon its axis. The arms must be kept bent just as seen in the cut, except at the extreme backward inclination, where they may be allowed to stretch out at their full length for a moment. As in all other similar exercises, the circling must be the same number of times each way.

Fig. 9. FINGER STRETCHED POSITION, *one, two, or three times.*

Rings at the height of the shoulders. One takes his position between them. He puts his hands through the rings, spreads the fingers out as far as possible, and brings their back surfaces against the upper part of the rings. Without changing the location of the feet, and with the body kept unbendingly straight, he makes an inclination backward as if he would permit himself to fall. The resistance against the loss of balance comes from the outstretched fingers, which must be so held as to press equally against the ring. This is a difficult exercise at first, but brings the extensors of the fingers into action as nothing else will.

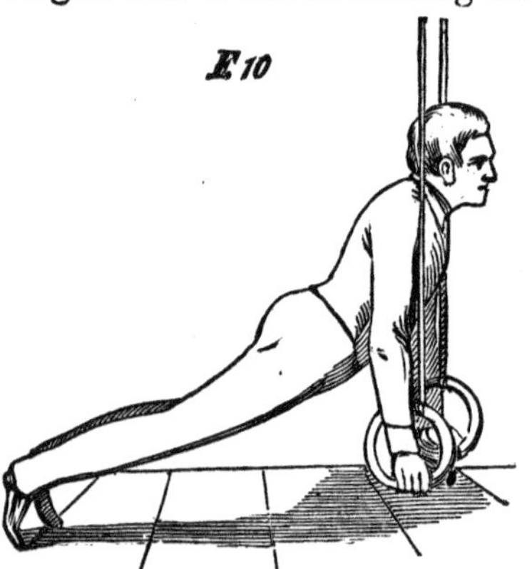

Fig. 10. CHEST STRETCHED POSITION, *during two, four, or six inhalations.*

Rings one foot from the floor. Grasp from the outside as shown in the cut, arms exactly perpendicular.

Legs straight, supported on the points of the toes. The rope must touch the shoulder. One hand can be lifted, and the weight of the body supported by one hand, though this exercise belongs to the second series.

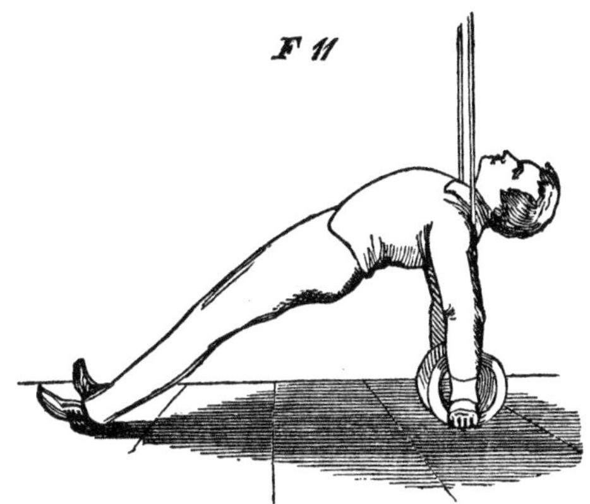

Fig. 11. BACK STRETCHED POSITION, *during two, four, or six inhalations.*

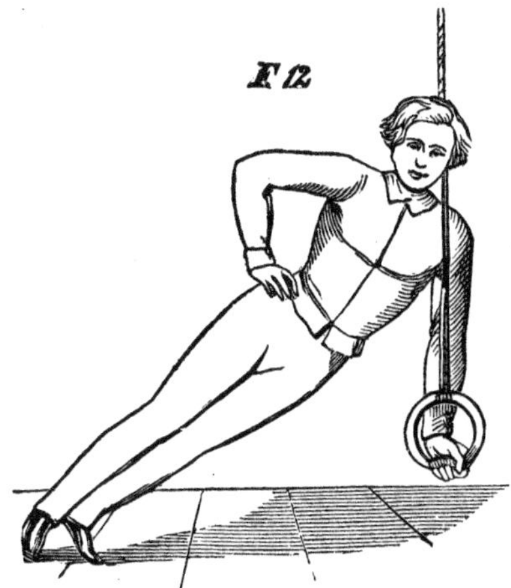

Rings same as in the last. Grasp with the spoke grasp from the outside, in such a manner that the rope is brought close behind the shoulder joint, and the shoulders braced against the rope. The ropes perpendicular, while the body is kept rigid, with the chest arched upward.

Fig. 12. SIDE STRETCH POSITION, *during two, four, or six inhalations.*

Ring still one foot from the floor. The hand seizes the ring on the outside with the spoke grasp, the rope touching the front of the shoulder. Arm exactly perpendicular. Body otherwise just as represented.

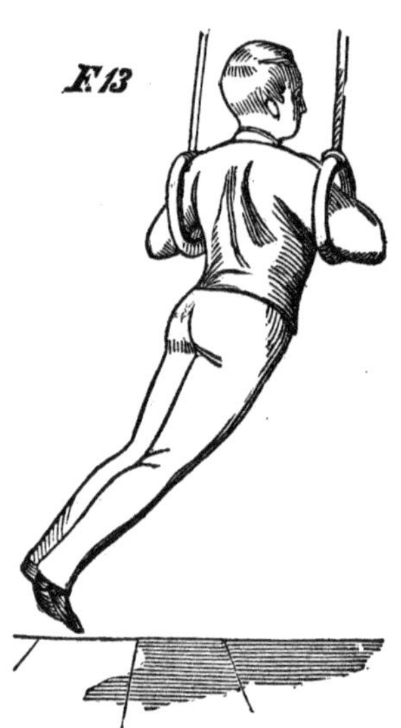

Fig. 13. ARM HANG, *during one, two, or three inhalations.*

Rings a little higher than the shoulders. Bend the forearm on the arm, and push the elbows through the ring as far as possible. Hold the body in the position shown in the cut. There should be no swinging.

Fig. 14. SUPPORT HANG, *during two, four, or six inhalations.*

Rings as high as the breast. Hands take hold from the outside with the support grasp. With a little spring the body can be lifted into the position seen in

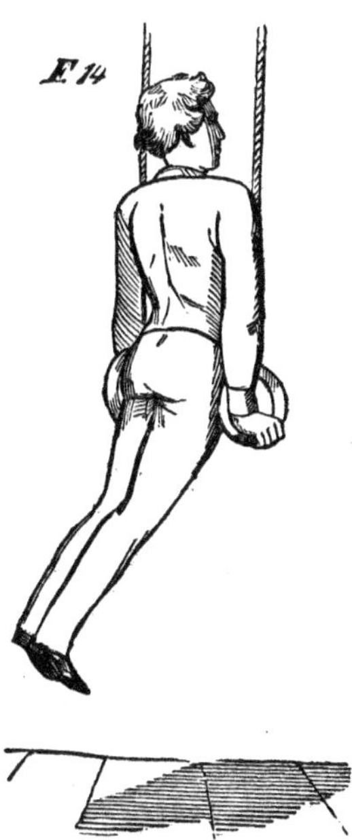

the cut. Beginners, with but little muscle, had better hang the rings no higher than the abdomen. Back straight and rigid. Chest arched forward. Feet locked. Body held still.

Fig. 15. Side Hanging, *with bending of the Hips, two, four, or six times.*

Height of the ring and position of the two arms, the feet and the hips are well shown. The hips are drawn upward and allowed to fall, as suggested in the dotted line.

Fig. 16. Perpendicular Foot Bending and Stretching, *from the Shoulder Hang, eight, twelve, or sixteen times.*

Rings as high as the head. Place the arms firmly in position and hold the body still. Toes are stretched

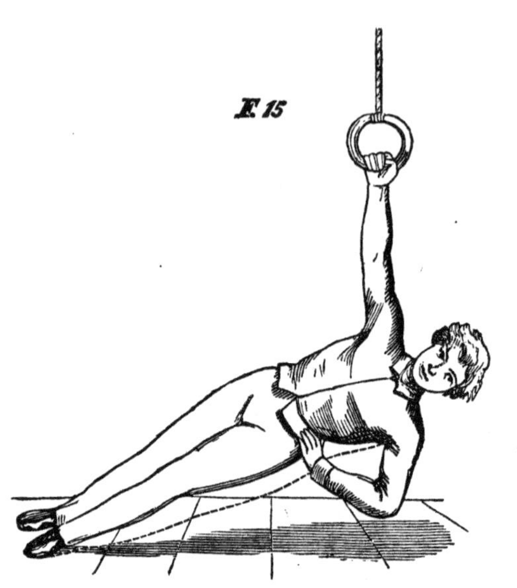

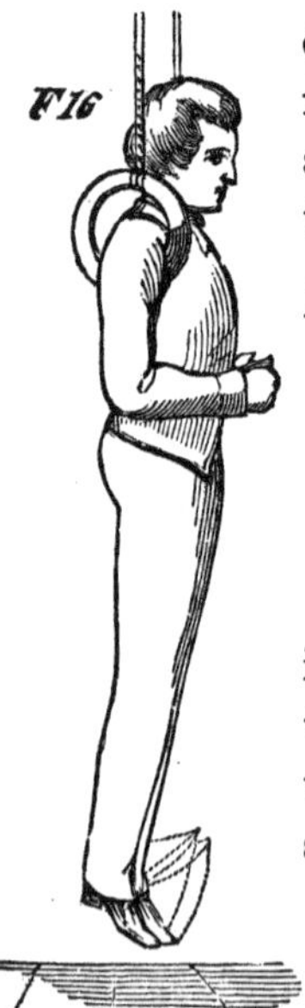

down as near the floor as possible, and drawn up near the ankle.

Fig. 17. Leg Twisting, *from the shoulder hang, eight, twelve, or sixteen times.*

Position same as in the last. Turn the toes slowly and vigorously outward and inward.

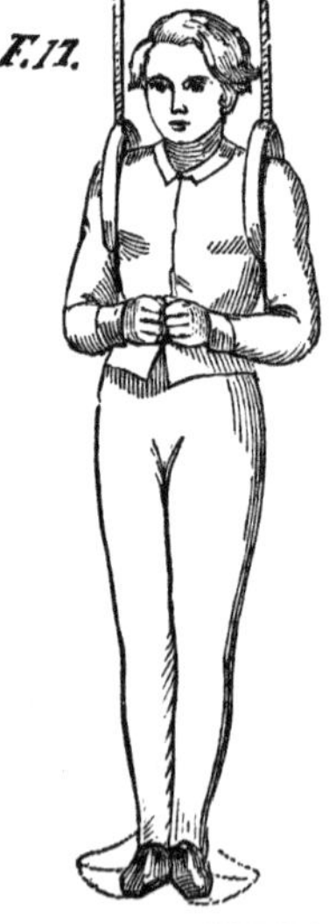

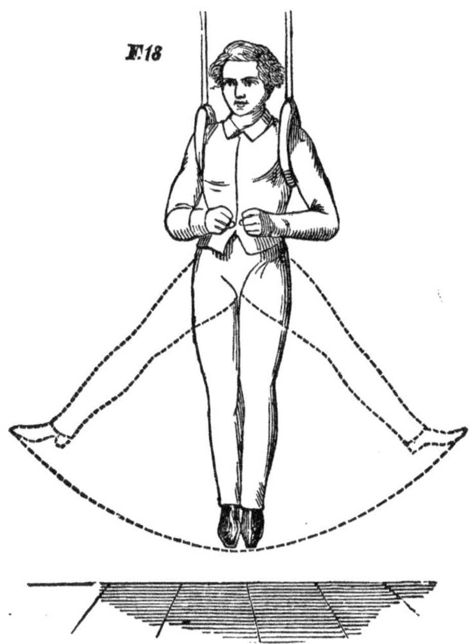

Fig. 18. LEG SPREADING, *from the Shoulder Hang.*

Position same as the last two exercises. The legs are thrown out exactly sidewise and with great vigor. The position of the feet when in contact and when separated is well shown.

Fig. 19. KNEE LIFTING, *from the Shoulder Hang.*

Rings in the same position. In this and the following three exercises, the hands seize the ropes close above the rings. By this means, a more concentrated exercise upon the corresponding muscles of the legs is secured. The knees are drawn up as high as possible. Those who are muscular and flexible, can carry the knees as high as the chest.

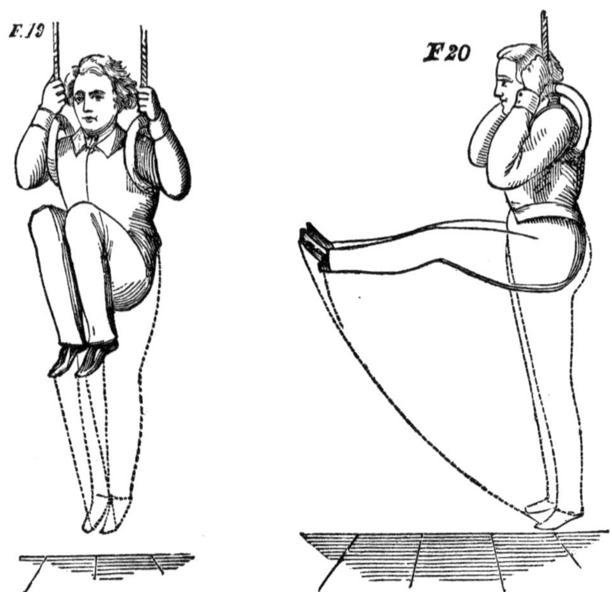

Fig. 20. HORIZONTAL LEG RAISING, *from the Shoulder Hang, two, four, or six times.*

Rings, hands and body in the same position as in *Fig.* 19. The legs are kept perfectly straight, and they are raised as shown in the figure where they are held for a moment.

Fig. 21. HORIZONTAL LEG SPREADING, *from the Shoulder Hang.*

The body and hands continue in the same position, except that here and in the next exercise the rings may be placed a little lower, perhaps as high as the shoulder. The legs are raised exactly as in the last, and being thus held they are carried apart as in the cut. Do not fail to keep the legs straight.

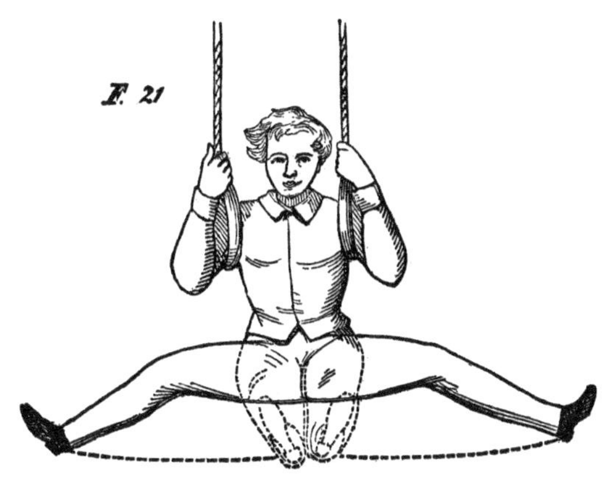

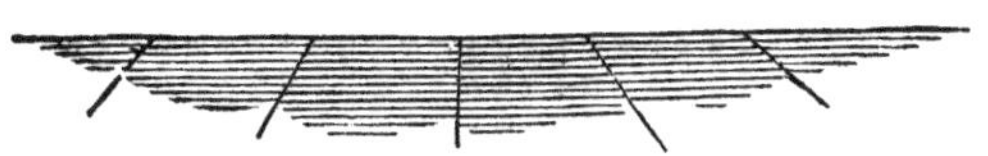

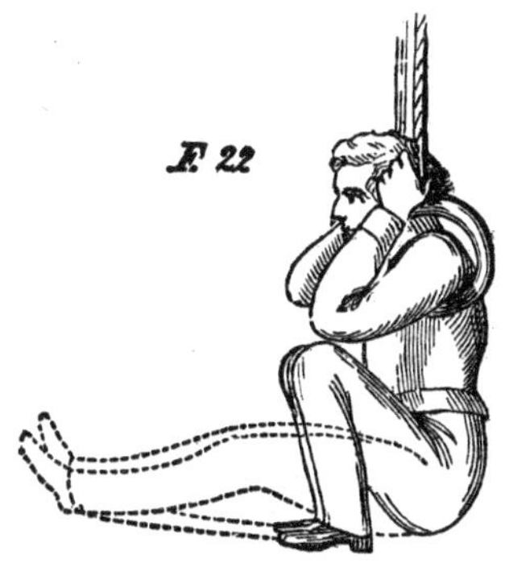

Fig. 22. KNEE EXERCISE, *from Horizontal position, two, three, or four times.*

Same position of the body and hands as in the last. Legs as in *Fig*. 20. Then they are bent at the knee to an acute angle and back again.

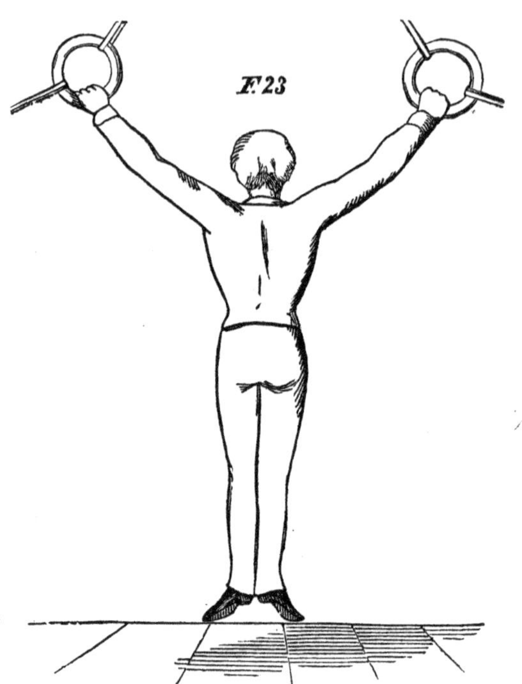

Fig. 23. SUSPENSION *from Spread Arms, six, eight, or ten inhalations.*

Rings sidewise, high enough to suspend the body from them. Head erect; back straight; legs straight and close together; feet at right angles.

Fig. 24. STIRRUP CROSSING, *four, six, eight times.*

Rings as high as the hips. Support grasp from the inside. Legs cross each other, so that each alternates before and behind the other. Hold the rings so that they will not partake of the movement. Count as one in this and similar exercises, the movements of both legs. It will be self evident, that to stand in the stirrups without movement, develops varied muscular

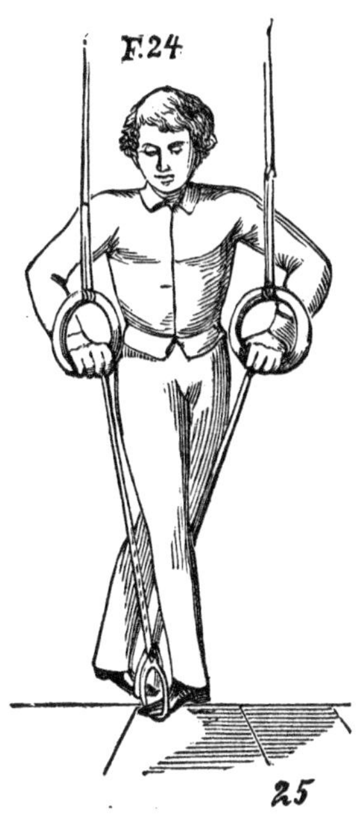

action in the legs and feet.

It will be observed that the toes only, rest upon the stirrups. For obvious reasons the feet should not be pushed through to the heels.

Fig. 25. STIRRUP SPREADING, *two, four, or six times.*

Rings as high as the waist. Support grasp from the outside. Move the legs sidewise rapidly. Keep the rings in their place.

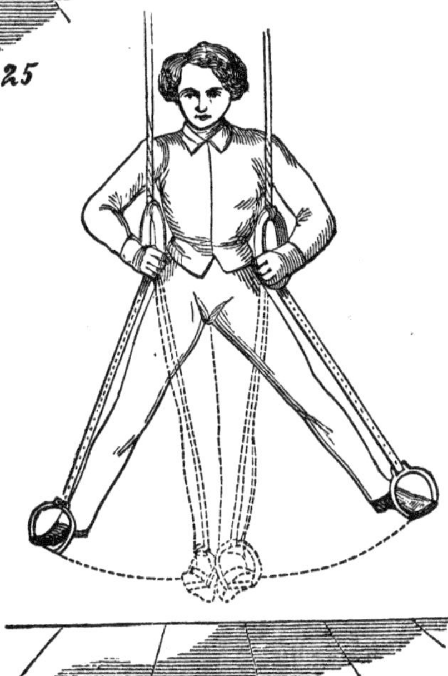

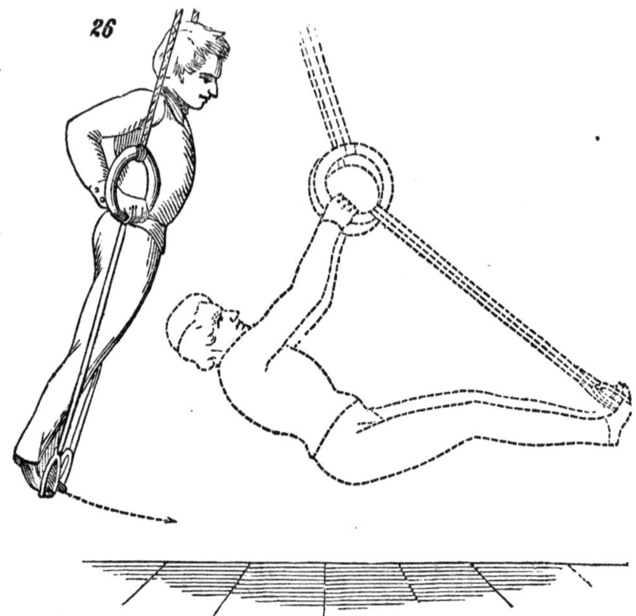

Fig. 26. SWINGING IN STIRRUPS, *four, eight, or twelve times.*

Rings as high as the waist or chest. Support grasp from the inside. Swing as upon any ordinary swing, when standing.

Fig. 27. SUSPENDED RUNNING IN THE STIRRUPS.

Rings and stirrups as in *Fig.* 26. Make the same motions of the legs as in running. As the legs pass each other they should be close together.

Fig. 28. STIRRUP STANDING INCLINATION, *in the Elbow Hang, four, six, or eight times.*

Standing in the stirrups, the rings are placed as high as the shoulder. Arms as seen in the cut. The body is thrown vigorously forward and backward.

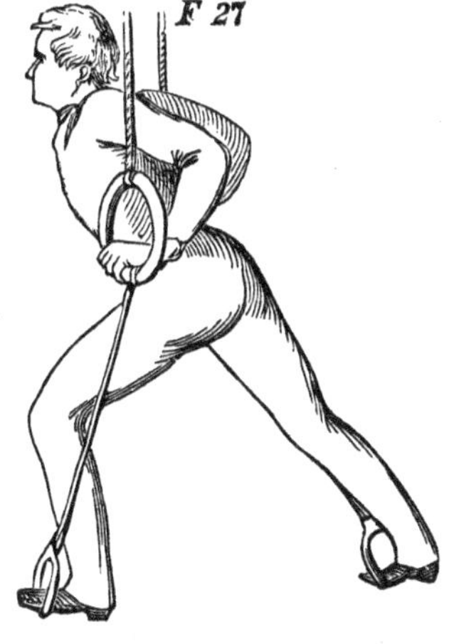

Fig. 29. SITTING DOWN IN THE STIRRUPS, *two, four, or six times.*

Standing in the stirrups, the rings are placed as high as the waist. Now sit down so as to touch the heels. In rising, use the legs alone, simply employing the arms to steady the body.

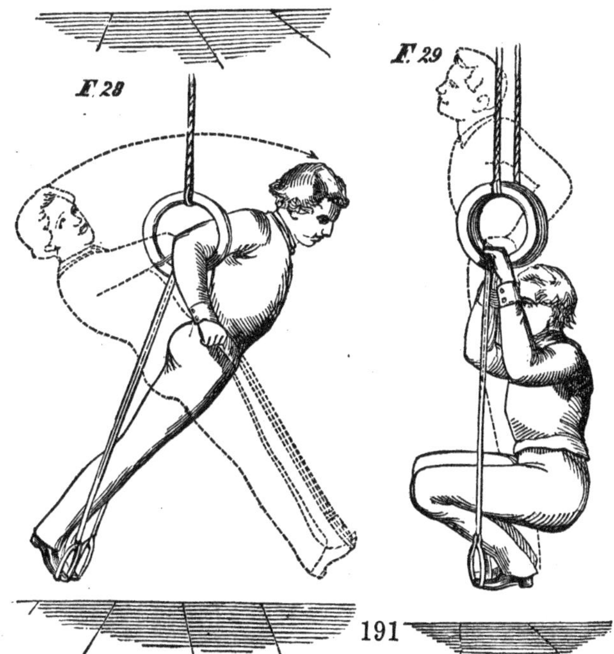

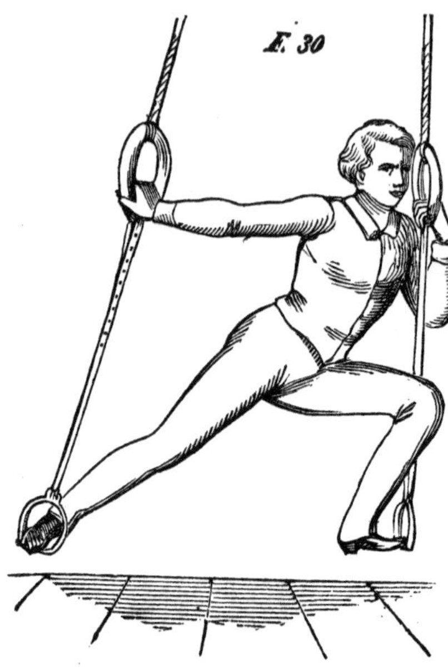

Fig. 30. KNEE CHARGING IN THE STIRRUPS, *four*, *six*, *or eight times*.

Standing in the stirrups, the rings are placed as high as the chest. Charge out on either side just as represented in the cut. Make the stride as great as possible.

SECOND SERIES.

Fig. 31. CHEST EXPANDING, WITH LETTING DOWN, *two*, *four*, *or six times*.

Rings at the lowest point. Arms perpendicular. Body straight; supported at the feet on the points of the toes, and with the hands seizing the rings as seen in the cut. Bend the elbows and let the body down slowly. Raise it again slowly. The arms do nearly all the labor.

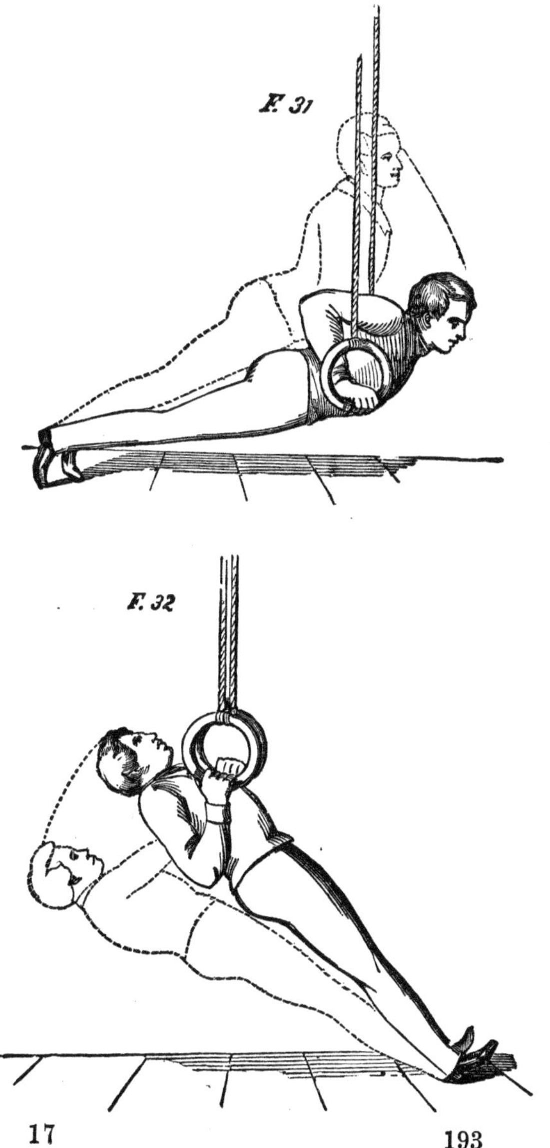
F. 31
F. 32

Fig. 32. HALF LYING, WITH LIFTING BY THE ARMS, *two, three, or four times.*

Rings as high as the chest. Seize the rings from the outside with the support grasp, and bring the body beneath the rings in an almost lying down position. Keep the body and neck in a straight line rigidly. Now draw the chest up to the rings, and let the body down again to the full length of the arms.

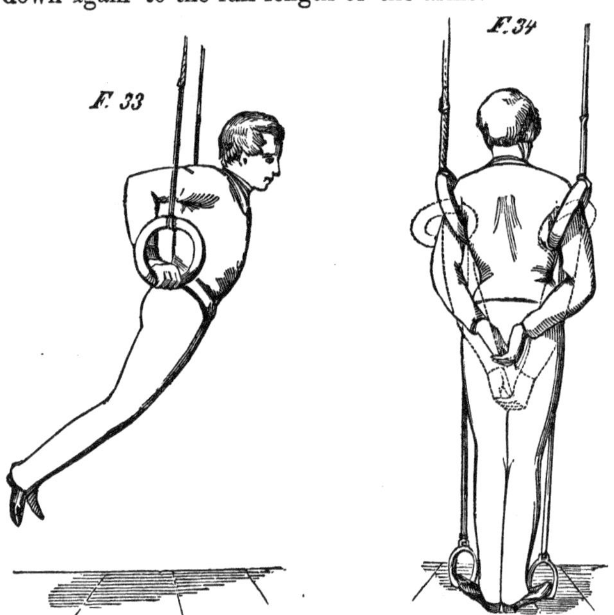

Fig. 33. ANGULAR SUPPORT HANGING, *during two, four, or six inhalations.*

Rings as high as the shoulders. Seize the rings from the inside with the support grasp, and spring into the position seen in *Fig.* 14; then let yourself slowly down into the position of *Fig.* 33. Head erect, chest thrown well forward, back straight, legs close together.

Fig. 34. DOWN THRUSTING OF THE LOCKED HANDS ON THE BACK, *four, six, or eight times.*

Rings as high as the shoulders. Stirrups touch the floor. Tips of the toes in the stirrups, heels together, and resting firmly on the floor. Arms thrust through the rings, and hands locked on the back. Thrust the hands downward, and draw the shoulders backward so that the tips of the toes will be raised by stirrups.

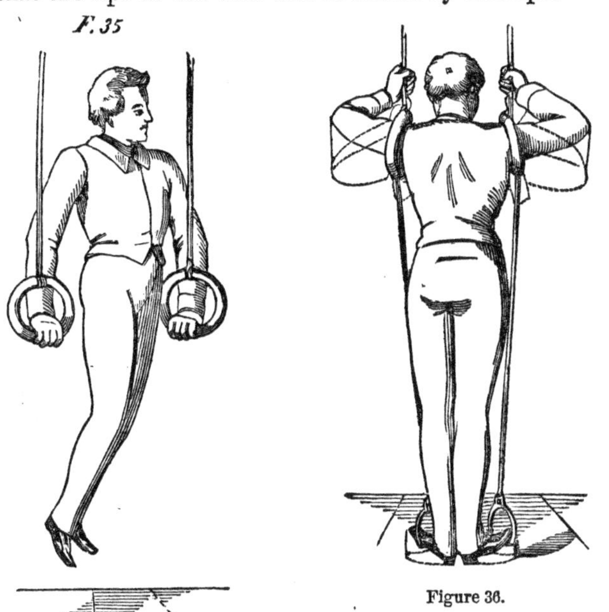

Figure 36.

Fig. 35. BODY TURNING IN THE SUPPORT HANG, *one, two, or three times.*

Rings at the waist. Seize the rings from the inside with the support grasp. The straightened body sustained by the hands is turned from side to side, the upper part one-eighth of a circle and the lower part one-fourth of a circle at each swing or turn.

Fig. 36. RING LIFTING BY THE SHOULDERS, *two, four, or eight times.*

Arms put through the rings, which then rest upon the shoulders. Stirrups reach the floor, toes are placed in them, hands grasp the ropes above the rings. Keep the heels firmly on the floor. Now by a vigorous raising of the shoulders you lift the stirrups, raising the toes until you draw the stirrups away from the toes altogether.

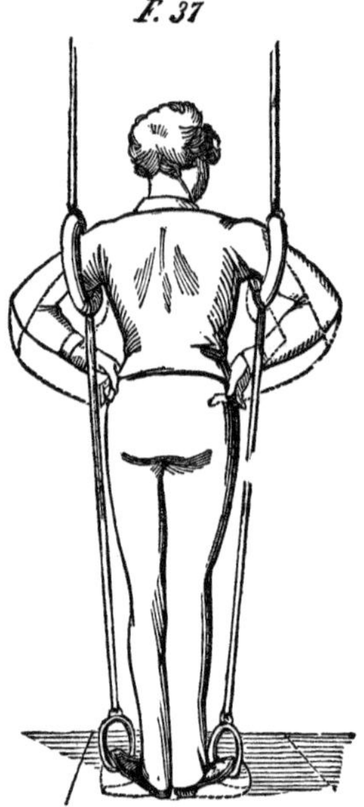

Fig. 37. RING LIFTING BY THE ARM, *two, four, or six times.*

This exercise is the same as the last, except that the rings are placed on the middle of the arm, and the principal exertion is in the lower part of the body which seeks to resist the tendency of the stirrups to slip off the feet.

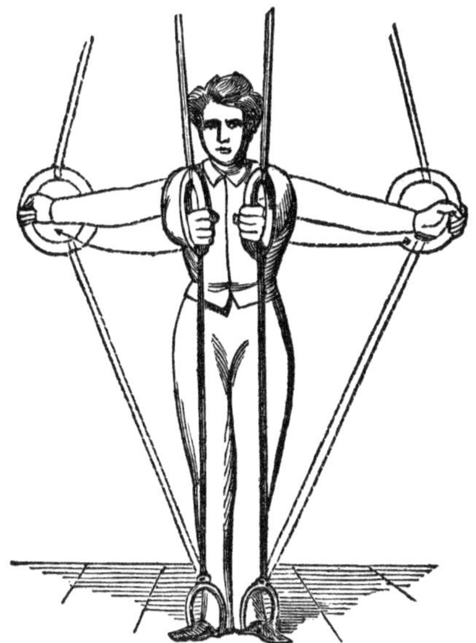

Figure 38.

Fig. 38. CHEST EXPANDING, *two, four, or six times.*

Rings as high as the chest. Adjust the stirrup straps so that when the rings are held out at arms length from the body, the stirrups will touch the floor. Put the feet into the stirrups as far as the heels. Take hold of the rings with the support grasp from the inside. Stretch out the arms in front of the body, and then, keeping the arms straight, carry them backward as far as possible. As soon as the straps are drawn tightly, the feet begin to offer a point of resistance, which may be increased to any desired degree. The body remains firm with heels upon the ground.

Fig. 39. BACK STRETCHING, *two, four, or six times.*

Rings and stirrups same as the last, with the legs

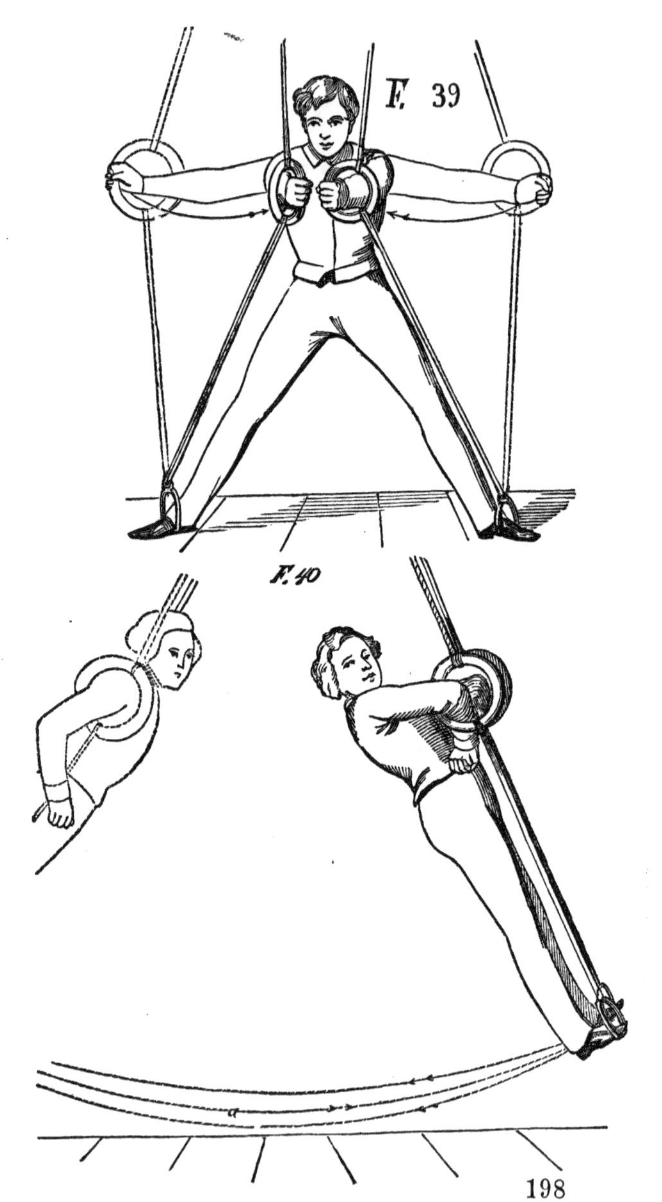
F. 39
F. 40
a

stretched apart. Hands seize the rings from the inside, (support grasp) and the arms are spread wide apart. They are kept straight, and brought together in front until they meet, overcoming as completely as possible the resistance offered by the feet. If the feet move, re-establish them before repeating the exercise.

Fig. 40. SHOULDER-ELBOW SWING IN THE STIRRUPS, *four, six, or eight times.*

Begin with the elbow-hang, the body inclined backward. Swing backward, sliding into the shoulder-hang. Swing forward and return to the elbow-hang. When swinging backward spread out the legs, and when you reach the extreme backward point bring the feet together again, and when swinging forward hold them together.

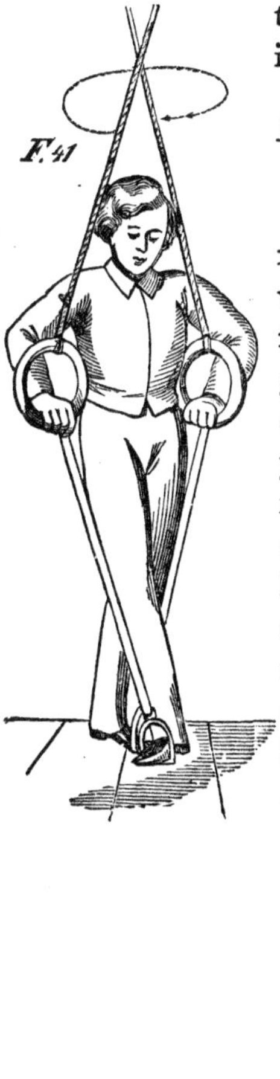

F. 41

Fig. 41. TWISTING SWING, *one, two, or three times.*

Standing in the stirrups, the rings should be as high as the waist. Take hold of the rings from the inside with the support grasp, and rotate the body on its own axis from side to side until you reach a semi-circle. As the ropes cross each other, the straps are made to cross each other likewise, through the action of the muscles of the legs. The rotation ought not to go beyond a semi-circle, else it may become irregular and injure the apparatus.

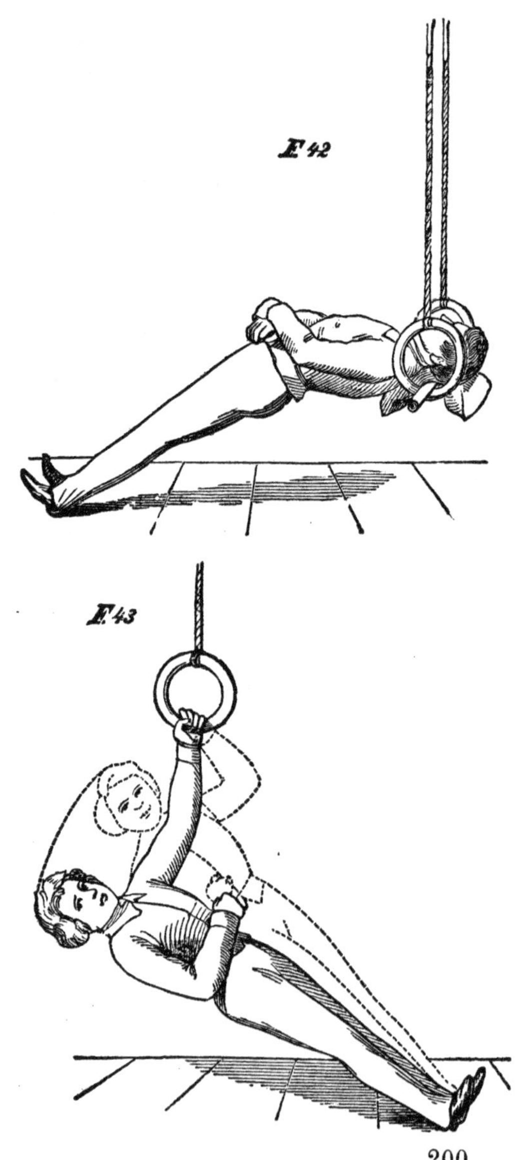
F. 42
F. 43

Fig. 42. NAPE BRACING POSITION, *during two, four, or six inhalations.*

The rings are placed at their lowest position, or within a foot of the floor. A strip of wood is placed in the rings, and upon it some soft object like a cushion or shawl. The back part of the head is laid upon the cushion and the heels touch the floor. The body is arched upward and held in that position.

Fig. 43. DRAWING UP BY ONE ARM IN THE BACK STRETCHING POSITION, *one, two, or three times.*

Rings as high as the head, though if the rings are placed a little lower, the action of the muscles will be greatly intensified. *The two heels must rest on the floor,*

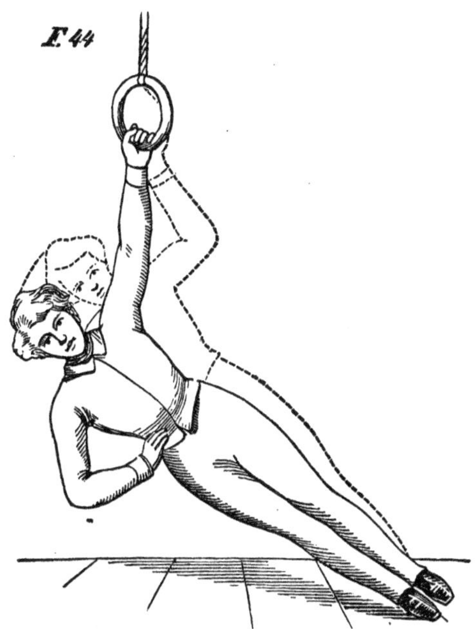

with the body nearly horizontal, and the arm straight.

The body is to be kept straight and stiff, while with the one arm it is drawn up as near as possible to the ring, and then it is let down as slowly as possible.

Fig. 44. DRAWING UP BY ONE ARM IN THE SIDE STRETCHING POSITION, *one, two, or three times.*

Position of the rings, arm and body same as in the last, except that in this, instead of the two heels resting on the floor, the *outside of the lower foot rests on the floor*. Holding the body straight, raise it without twisting, to the ring, and let it down slowly.

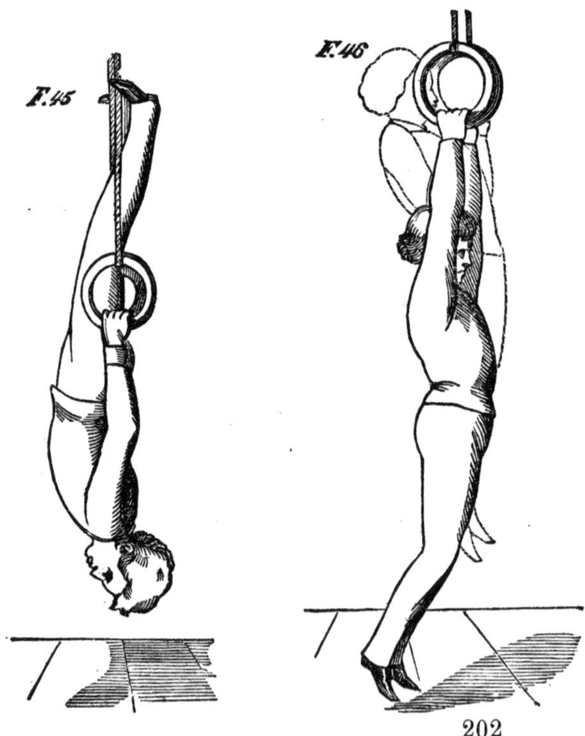

Fig. 45. PERPENDICULAR SUPPORT, HEAD DOWNWARD, *during two, three, or four inhalations.*

Rings as high as the head. Seize from the outside with the hand grasp. Spring from the floor and turn a half summerset, reaching the inverted position. Each leg should rest against the rope on its own side, the rope being inside the ankle. The body must be kept straight.

Fig. 46. PERPENDICULAR BODY LIFTING WITH THE TWO ARMS, *two, three, or four times.*

Rings as high as you can reach. Seize from the outside with the hang grasp. Keep the body straight, and draw the head up as high as the rings, letting it down slowly.

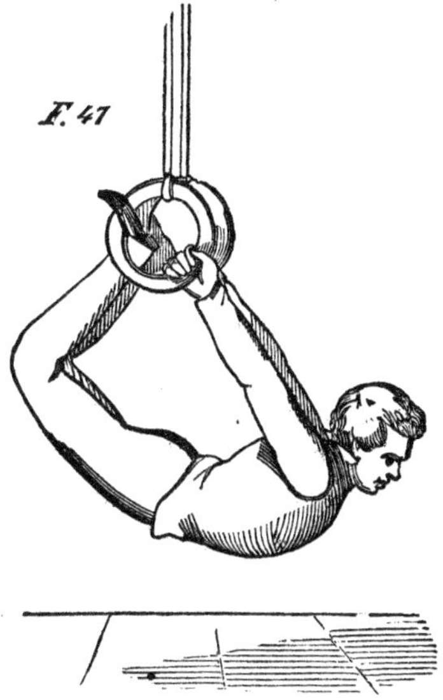

Fig. 47. HAND AND FOOT HANGING, *during one, two, or three inhalations.*

Rings are placed and grasped as in *Fig*. 45. Commence the exercise likewise in the same manner; but when the body reaches the turning point, put the toes in the rings. Bend the knees and body as seen in the cut.

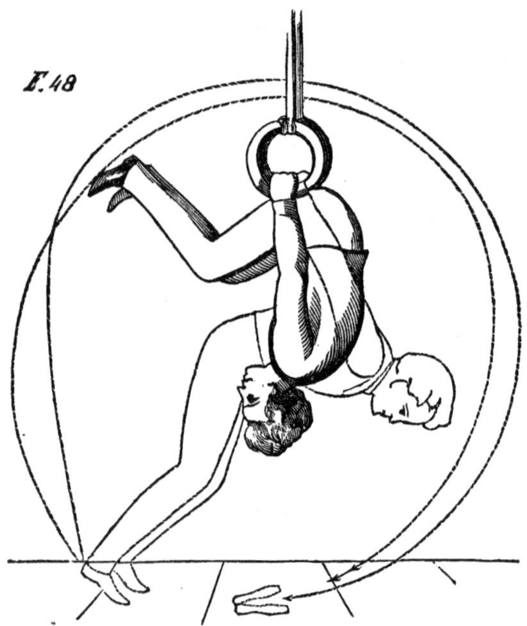

Fig. 48. SUMMERSET FORWARD AND BACKWARD, *one, two, or three times.*

Rings as high as the head or shoulders. The first half of the movement is exactly like that in *Figs*. 45 and 47; but unlike those, this one is completed. Turning completely over thus forward, immediately reverse and turn backward.

Fig. 49. ANGULAR SUPPORT DRAWING, *two, three, or four times.*

Rings at shoulder height, lift yourself into the position seen in *Fig.* 14. Keep your back and legs straight and rigid, and lower and raise yourself as seen in *Fig.* 49.

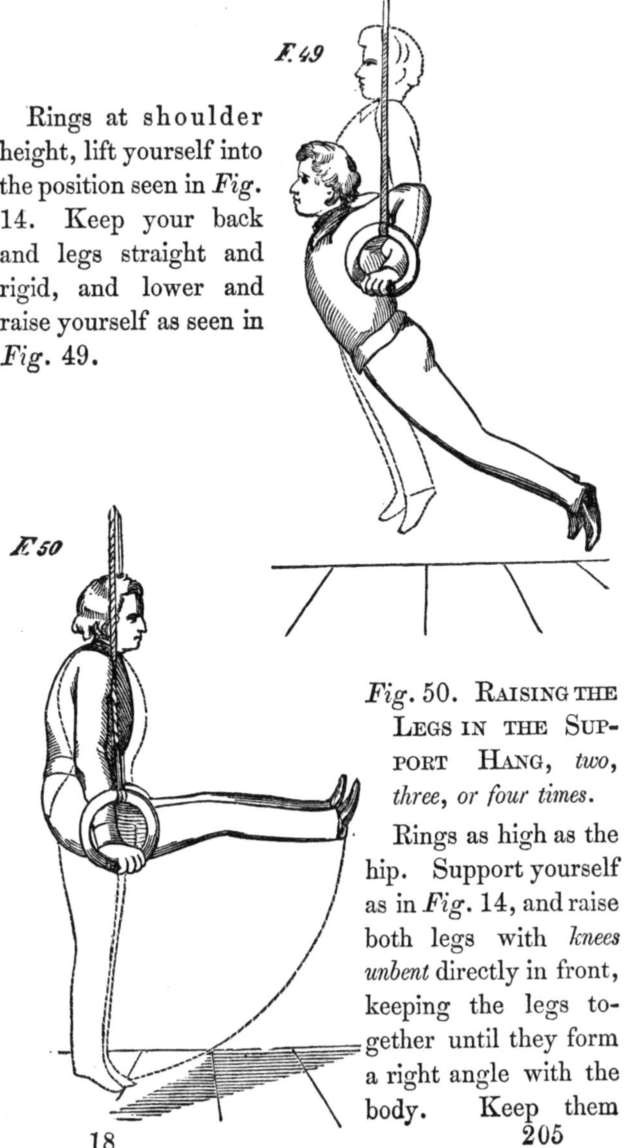

Fig. 50. RAISING THE LEGS IN THE SUPPORT HANG, *two, three, or four times.*

Rings as high as the hip. Support yourself as in *Fig.* 14, and raise both legs with *knees unbent* directly in front, keeping the legs together until they form a right angle with the body. Keep them while counting ten, and then let them down slowly.

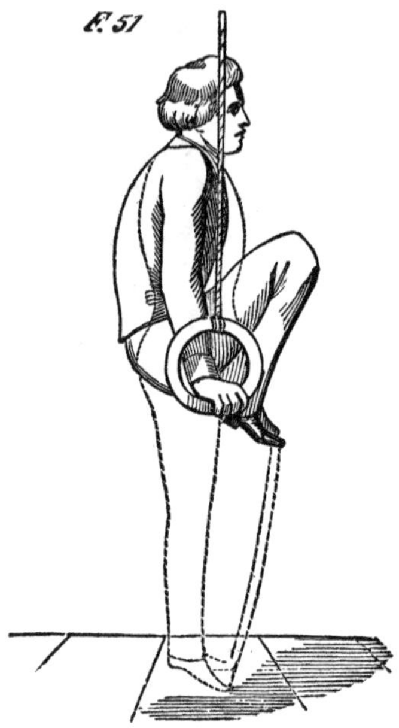

Fig. 51. Knee Raising in the Support Hang, *three, four, or five times.*

Rings, body, etc., as in the last. Raise the knees as high as possible, then thrust them down again with great force.

Fig. 52. Horizontal Leg Spreading in the Support Hang, *two, three, or four times.*

Preparation and position same as in *Fig*. 50. Spread the legs as far as possible directly sidewise. Do not touch the floor between the spreadings.

Fig. 53. Horizontal Leg Stretching from the Support Hang, *two, three, or four times.*

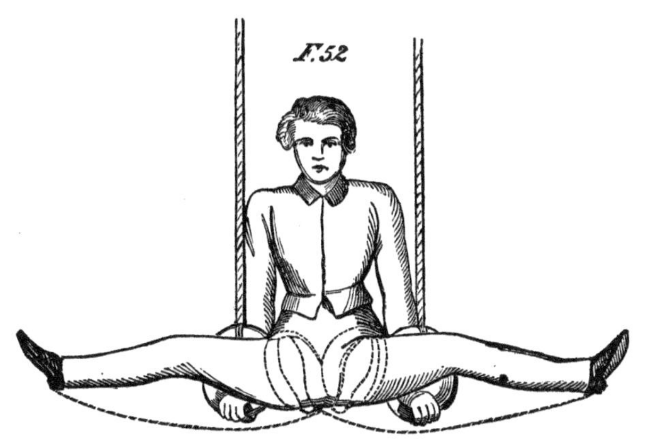

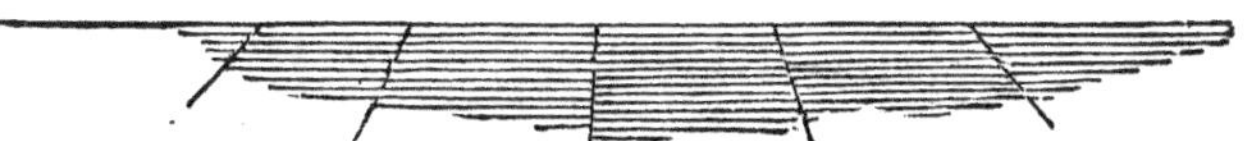

When the legs have been brought into the position of *Fig.* 51, thrust them out forcibly into the position of *Fig.* 50. When thrust out make sure there is no bend of the knee.

Fig. 54. HEAD DOWNWARDS, FEET FREE, *during four, six, or eight inhalations.*

In this exercise one proceeds as in *Fig.* 45, except the feet and legs do not touch the ropes. The body is kept suspended between the ropes as indicated in *Fig.* 54. Care must be exercised that the rings do not swing in the slightest degree.

Fig. 55. FALL HANG IN THE STIRRUPS, *four, eight, or twelve times.*

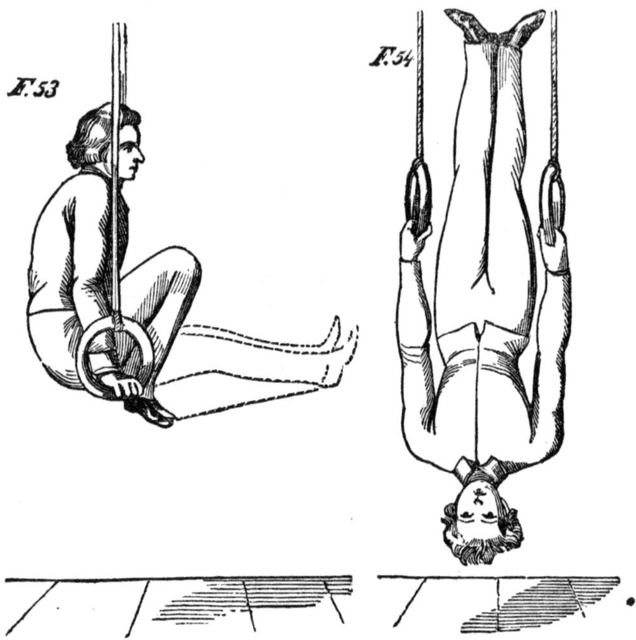

Rings as high as the chest. Stirrups so they will swing clear of the floor. Seize the rings from the inside with the support grasp. One throws himself forward between the rings, with the back stretched so that a curve is formed by the body from the head to the heels, and the arms are parallel with the straps. Now by an exertion of the arms the body is thrown back between the ropes, and into an opposite and reversed position. This time the rings are suspended sidewise over the front of the body.

In making this transition, the hang grasp with elbows beneath the hands is changed into the support grasp, with the elbows above the hands. This is partly accomplished through an upward action of the

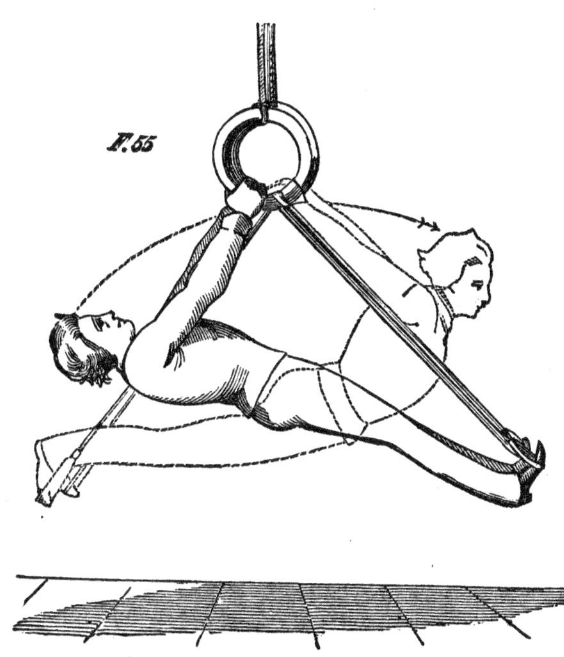

elbow, and partly through the turning of the rings, the firm grasp upon which is never relaxed. When going forward, one must pay close attention to the position of the elbows, as the arm and hand rotation may be a pronatory instead of a supinatory movement, in which case the front position would be entirely different from the one intended. This latter point is important.

Fig. 56. Bow Bracing Hang, *two, four, or six times.*

Standing in the stirrups the rings are chest high, and are grasped from the outside with the hang grasp. From the penpendicular stretched position one lets the

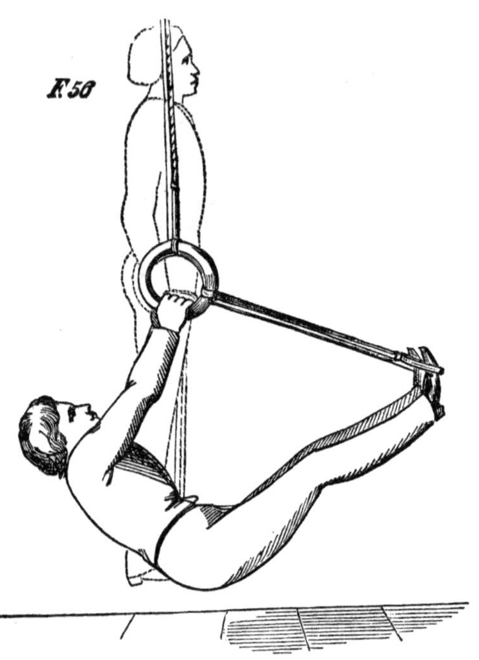

body fall backward until he reaches the position seen in the figure. In returning to the perpendicular position one uses only the arms.

Fig. 57. FALLING SIDEWISE IN STIRRUPS, *two, three, or four times.*

With rings at chest height when standing in the stirrups, they are from the outside grasped with the hang grasp. The straightened body lets itself down in a sidewise direction, both rings before the chest, accompanied by an inclination of the whole weight of the body in that direction. Thence with a drawing-in exertion of both arms he goes into the same position on the other side.

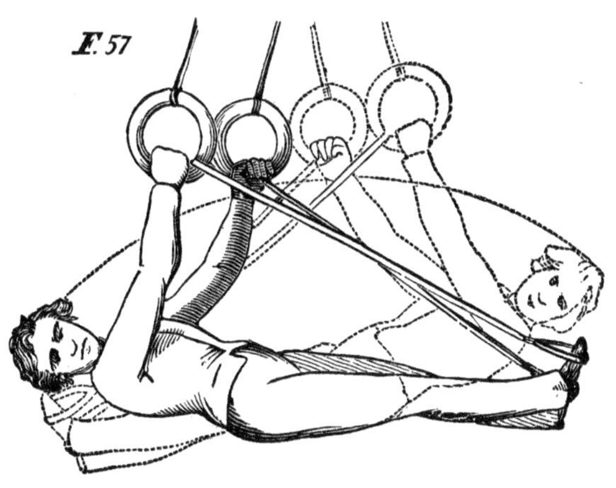

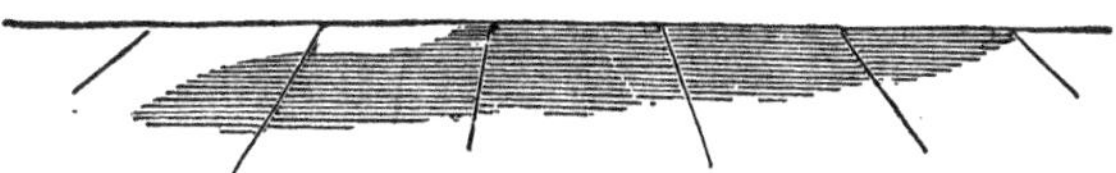

Fig. 58. STIRRUP CROSSING WITH HAND RESISTANCE, *two, three, or four times.*

Measured from the stirrups the rings are at shoulder height. Grasp them from the inside with the support grasp, and hold them as far apart as possible, while the legs which are standing in the stirrups, alternately cross each other in front as far as possible, the points of the feet being turned outward. The crossing forward and backward are counted but one. The resistance between the arms and legs can be increased ad libitum.

Fig. 59. STANDING INCLINATION IN THE SPREAD OUT GRASP, *two, four, or six times.*

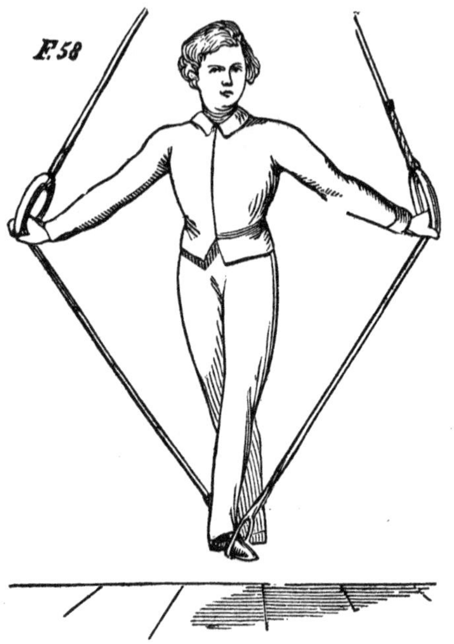

The rings which are fastened so as to be far apart from each other, are so high that one is just able to grasp them. They are taken with the hang grasp from the inside, one standing erect midway between them. Without changing the position of the feet, one inclines himself forward and then backward.

In moving forward, one must with muscular activity, keep perfect control over the movement and attitude, to make sure that it does not degenerate into a mere passive stretching of the body. The transition from one to the other position must not be accompanied with a swinging movement.

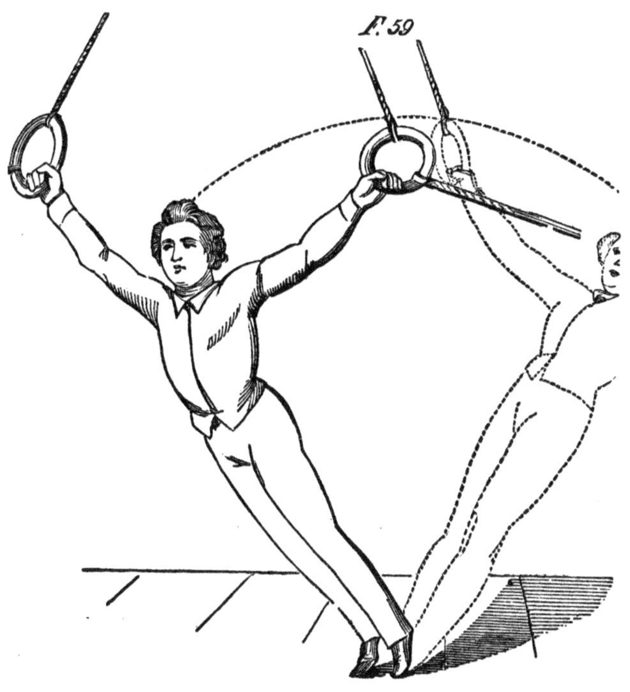

THIRD SERIES.

Fig. 60. FORWARD AND BACKWARD SWING WITH DRAWING UP, *two, three, or four times.*

The rings, at the highest grasp position, are seized from the outside with the hang grasp, and the pupil swings back and forth. In either direction, when the

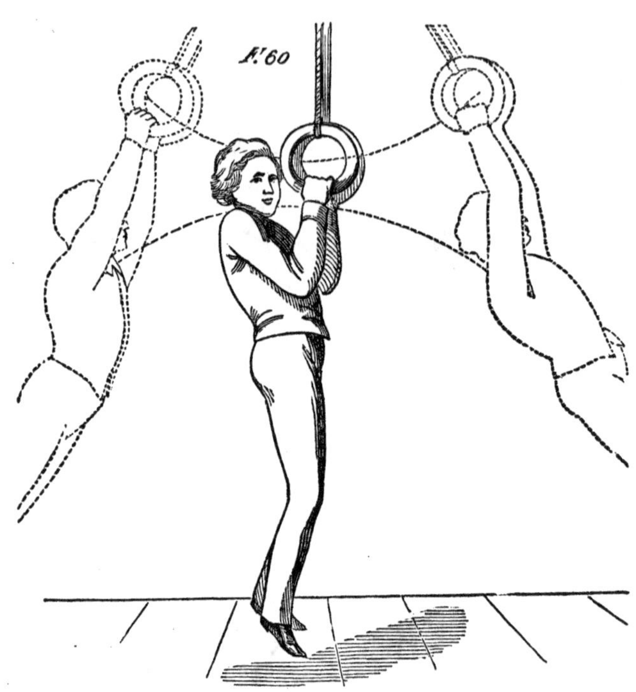

centre of the swing is reached, the body is drawn up by the arms, and at each end of the swing it is let down again to the full length of the arms.

Fig. 61. SIDEWISE SWING WITH DRAWING UP, *two, three, or four times.*

Position and grasping same as in *Fig.* 60. The swing takes place in an exactly sidewise direction. As before, the body is drawn up as near as possible to the rings, at the centre of each swinging, and let down again at the end points. On account of the sidewise position, the outer arm cannot attain the same straight attitude as the inner arm.

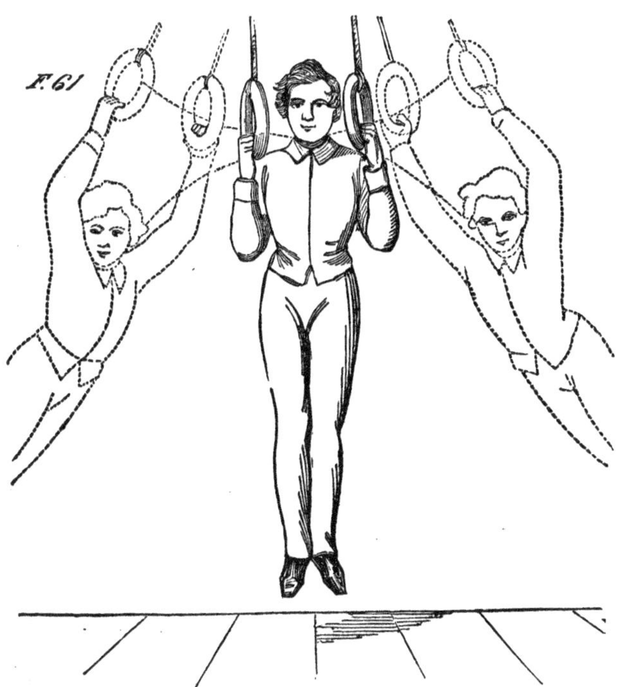

Fig. 62. ONE ARM HAND SWINGING, *two*, *four*, *or six times*.

The rings as before; one arm at a time grasps a ring. With the points of the feet one brings himself into a swinging movement, which is kept free from twisting or turning.

Fig. 63. BODY TWISTING WHEN SUSPENDED WITH THE HEAD DOWNWARD, *two*, *three*, *or four times*.

Assume the position in the figure, with the head just clearing the floor. If one has perfect control of the body he may raise himself higher. As soon as the body is firmly fixed in the illustrated position, the twisting commences, the body turning on its own axis a full quarter towards each side.

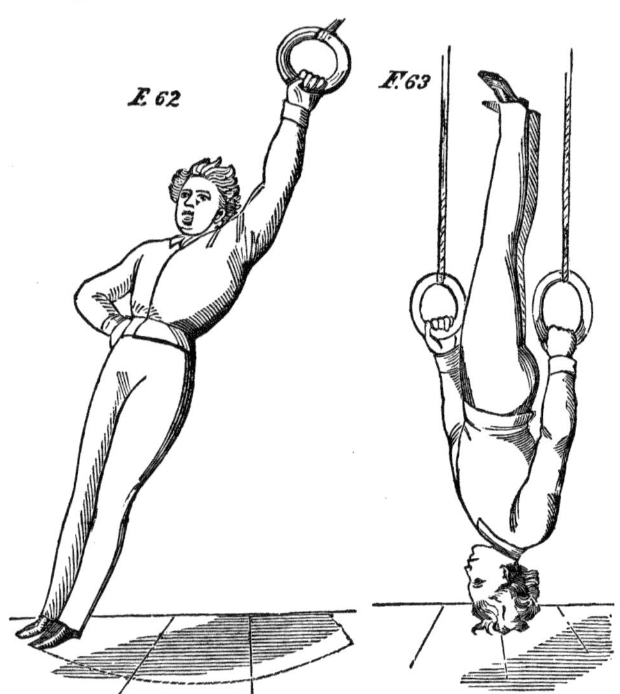

Fig. 64. SUSPENDED SUMMERSET, *two, three, or four times.*

In this exercise one proceeds as in *Fig.* 48, with the exception that here one's feet do not touch the ground; and to secure this, the rings are placed somewhat higher. Both the forward and backward summerset are executed without the assistance of a spring from the floor. The backward summerset commences from the drawn-in hang position. One must go down backwards as low as possible, so far that the knees are suspended perpendicularly between the rings over the floor.

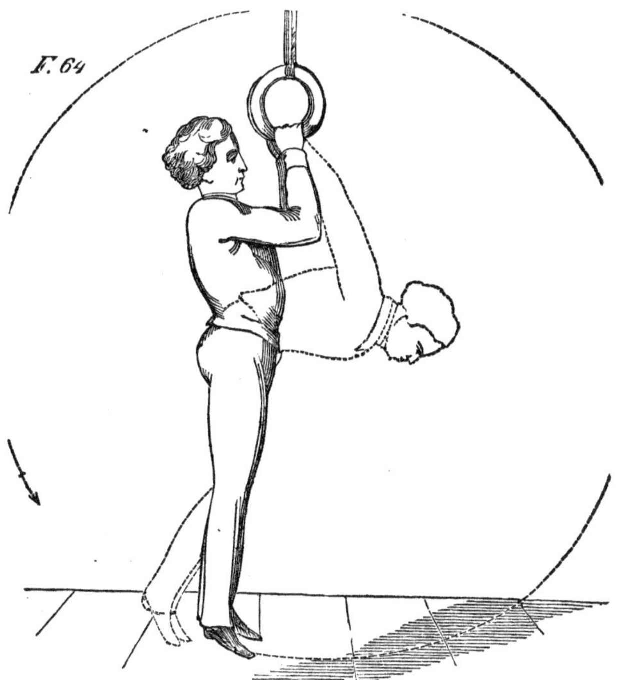

Fig. 65. Knee Bend Hanging, *one, two, or three times.*

Rings at head height, and from one to the other a strong wooden pole about three feet long is laid. To reach the position stand beneath the rings with the back stooped. Bend the hands backward and grasp the rings by the side of the pole. With a slight leap the legs are carried over the pole, and the hands let go. One leg after the other is now raised for a little time. In this way is measured the number of repetitions. In this case as in all others where there is an alternation between the two legs, or arms or sides of the body, the two are counted for one. At the close of this exercise, the head and upper part of the body rise up to grasp the rings again. The stirrup straps are left suspended, as a means of support in case the rings are not at once reached.

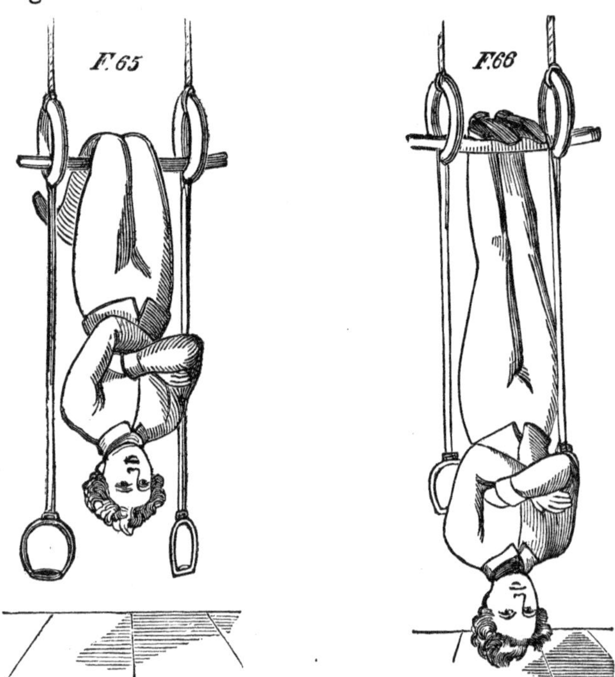

Fig. 66. Foot Point Hang, *during one, two, or three inhalations.*

Place the pole in the rings a little higher than the head. As in *Fig.* 48, the leap is made as for a summerset. The point of support is where the toes join the foot. The feet being placed on the pole, the hands leave the rings, and the body hangs straight.

The stirrup straps are allowed to remain so that in attempting to reach the rings with the hands, they may be resorted to if necessary.

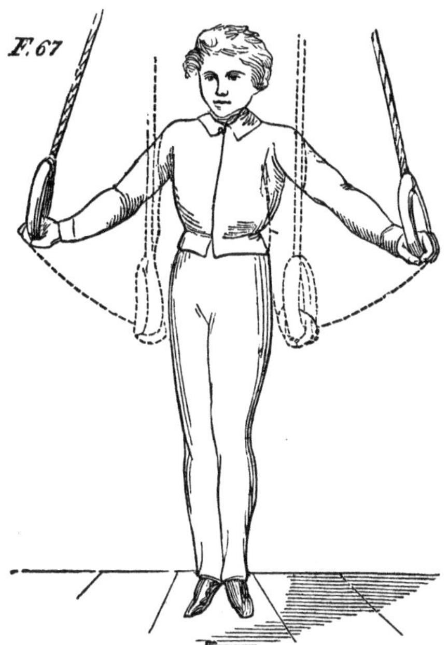

Fig. 67. ARM SPREADING IN THE SUPPORT HANG, *one, two, or three times.*

Rings as high as the shoulders. Leap into the simple support hang. Now move the arms sidewise very slowly as far as possible from the body, and then draw them back again with the same deliberation.

Fig. 68. CURVED SUPPORT HANG, *during one, two, or three inhalations.*

Rings as high as the shoulders, are grasped from the outside with the support grasp, in such a manner that the ropes rest behind the upper part of the arm and

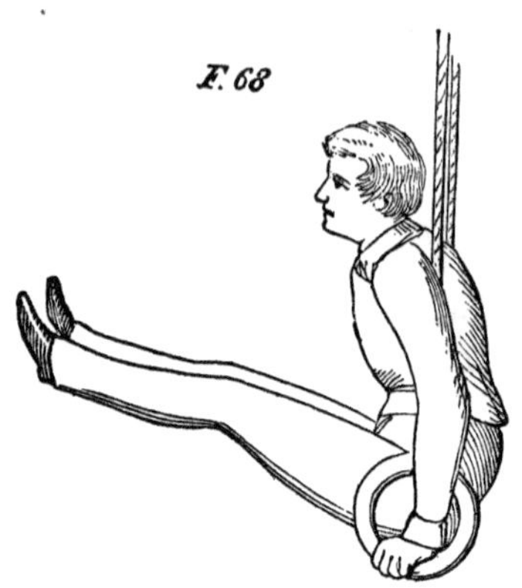

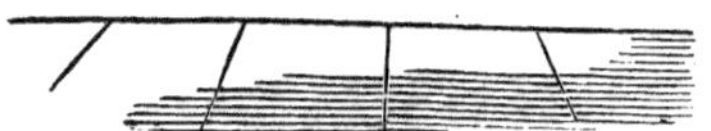

shoulder. By a slight bending of the elbows, one lets himself down a little. Now one raises his straight legs until they are above the horizontal line. The shoulders should lean firmly back against the ropes.

Fig. 69. ANGULAR SUPPORT SWING, *two, three, or four times.*

From the angular support hang, (*Fig.* 33.) one performs the swing by an effort of the legs. While swinging, the body may be raised and lowered by an effort of the arms.

Fig. 70. UNEQUAL SUPPORT CHANGE, *one, two, or three times.*

Rings at shoulder height. One is grasped from the outside with the hang grasp, and the other from the

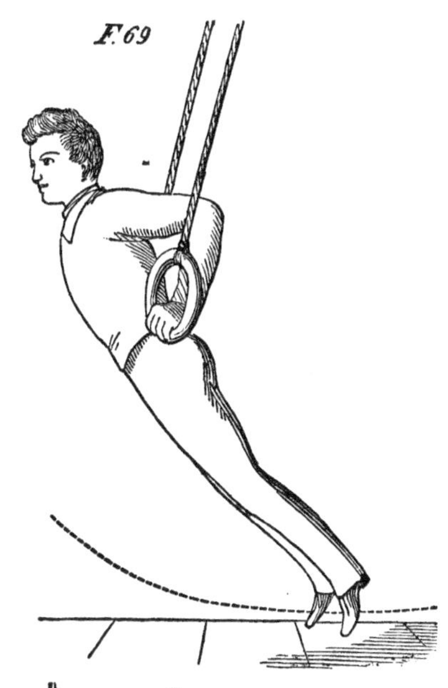

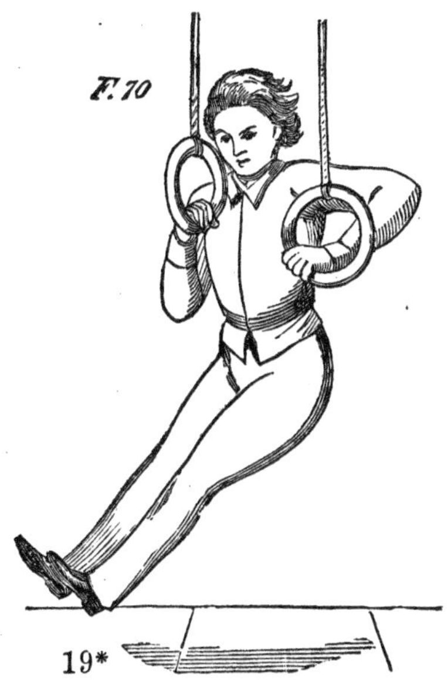

inside with the sup port grasp. As soon as the feet are lifted from the ground the changing begins. Each arm assumes as it may, at one time the angular support hang, and then the drawn-up hang. This alternating must take place without a swinging movement, and without having the feet touch the ground.

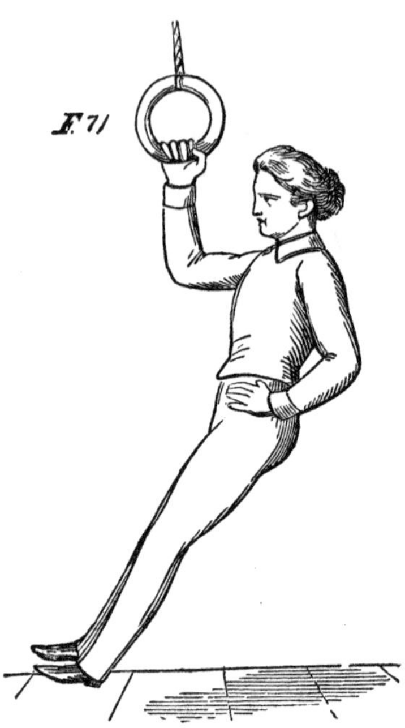

Fig. 71. ONE ARM DRAWN-IN HANG, IN THE STANDING UP POSITION, *one, two, or three times*.

Rings as high as the head. Grasp from the outside with the hang grasp. Alternate between the right and left arm. (It is perhaps always best, except in the case of left-handed people, to give the left hand and arm a little more than half the work, where this is possible. To secure this, many persons have arranged the apparatus with which the rings are raised and lowered, so that the left hand ring is always a little the higher.) Leaping slightly from the floor one goes into the position seen in the cut, in which he remains for a short time

This exercise differs from *Fig*. 80 in the downward

attitude of the legs, and from *Fig*. 83 in having the assistance of the leap from the floor.

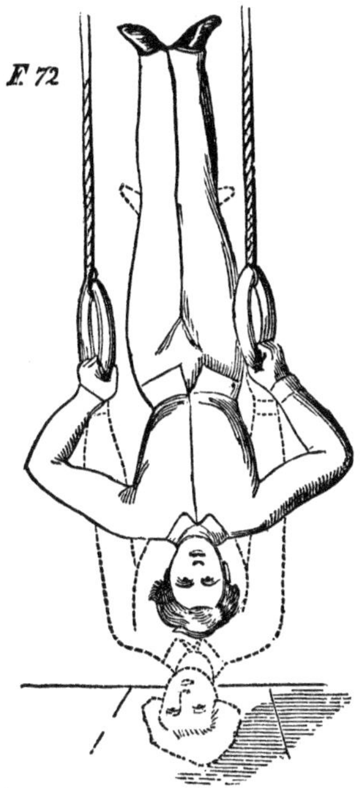

Fig. 72. Drawing Up in the Inverted Position, *two, three, or four times.*

As in *Fig*. 54, one goes into the inverted position, where the body is kept freely suspended between the arms and rings. From this position one keeps the body as straight as he can and draws it as high as possible. Then it is gradually lowered again. This is all to be done with the greatest deliberation, and without jerking or jolting.

Fig. 73. Drawing Up with the Spread Out Grasp, *one, two, or three times.*

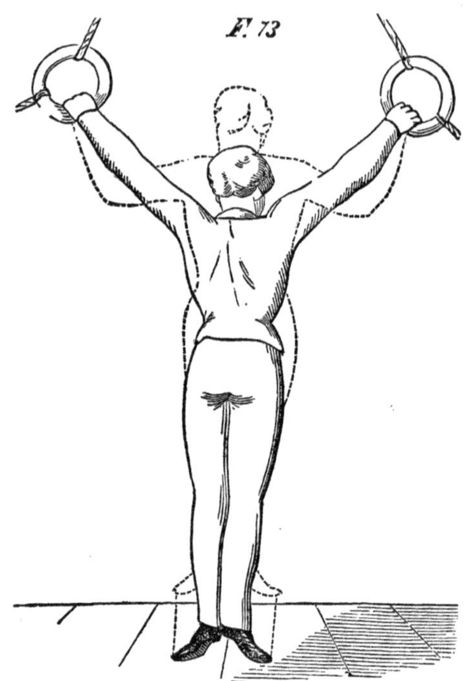

Position same as in *Fig.* 23. Then raise the body as high as possible with the arms, keeping the body straight between the two rings. Motions very slow.

Fig. 74. STRETCHED ANGULAR SUPPORT HANG, *one, two, or three times.*

With rings at shoulder height, one goes into the position of the angular support hang of *Fig.* 33. Now push one of the rings as far as possible from the body sidewise. The arm which remains in the angular support hang sustains the principal part of the weight of the body. With a lifting movement the body is gently and deliberately returned to the angular support hang, and carried to the other side. The feet are not

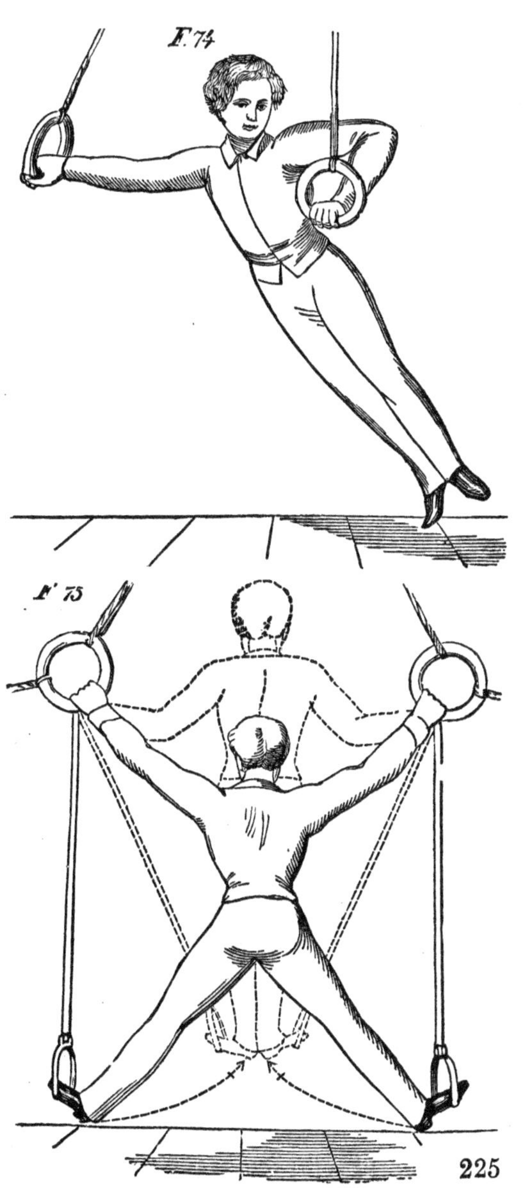
F. 74
F. 75

to touch the ground. If the movements are not executed very slowly, there will be a sidewise swinging of the body, which will greatly increase the difficulties.

Fig. 75. SPREAD OUT HANG WITH DRAWING TOGETHER OF THE LEGS, *three*, *four*, *or five times*.

The rings are fixed by the side ropes at head height. The stirrups are at a length which permits the legs to take a fall, though not an exaggerated spread apart position. Each hand grasps a ring, each foot is placed in a stirrup. The feet are then drawn together until the heels touch.

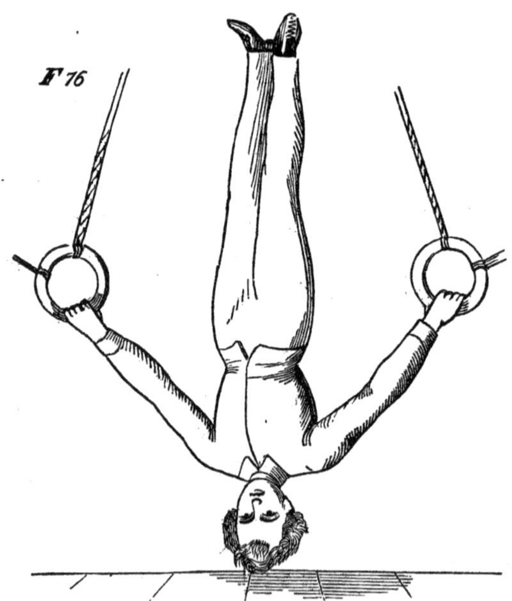

Fig. 76. HEAD DOWN IN THE SPREAD HANG, *during two*, *three*, *or four inhalations*.

The rings are attached at the side and raised to the

highest grasp point; (they are placed too low in the cut,) one remains a moment in the simple spread out hang position, with feet off the ground, in order to concentrate the power upon the half summerset which is to follow. As soon as the body has reached the perpendicular line, midway between the rings, it is stretched out and kept straight in the inverted position.

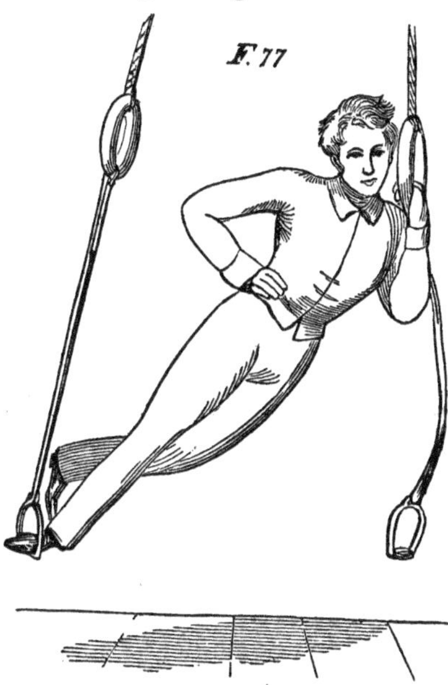

Fig. 77. DIAGONAL ATTITUDE, *two, three, or four times.*

Standing in the stirrups the rings are at chest height. With left hand, grasp the ring from the outside with hang grasp, and place the right foot in the opposite stirrup, whilst the free arm and leg are kept in the passive condition, and the body is kept straight. Follow the same rule with the other arm and leg.

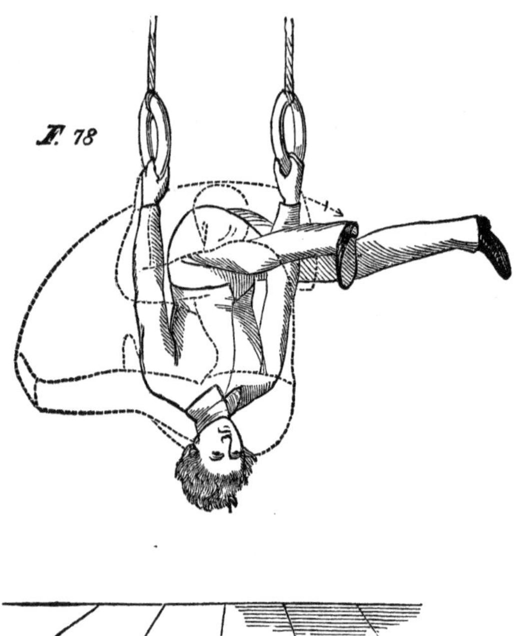

Fig. 78. SUMMERSET HANG IN A SIDEWISE DIRECTION, *two, three, or four times.*

From the drawn-in position with arms bent at a right angle, and with legs bent at a right angle to the body, somewhat separated and at the same time straight, (similar to the position in *Fig.* 80. but now with both arms,) execute a summerset in a sidewise direction as far over as is permitted by the arm which comes between the legs. Alternate with the other side without touching the floor meanwhile.

Fig. 79. DRAWING UP AND SUPPORT CHANGING, *one, two, or three times.*

With rings a little above head height, one goes from

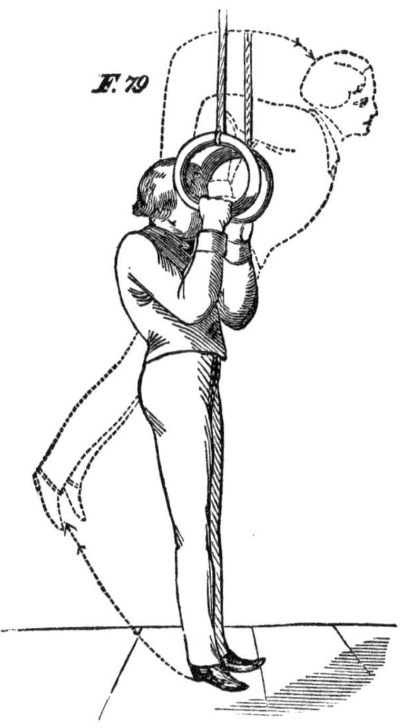

the drawn-up hang position of *Fig.* 46, through a drawing up, and back of the arms into the angular support hang, (*Fig.* 79,) and from that back again to *Fig.* 46. This is achieved without touching the floor. The rings must be turned round during the exercise, on account of the changes in position which naturally occur between the hang grasp and the support grasp.

Fig. 80. Drawing-up Hang with One Arm, in the Sitting Attitude, *one, two, or three times.*

Rings as high as the head. Hang grasp from the outside; both arms are now drawn up until bent at a right angle; then both legs are straightened and drawn

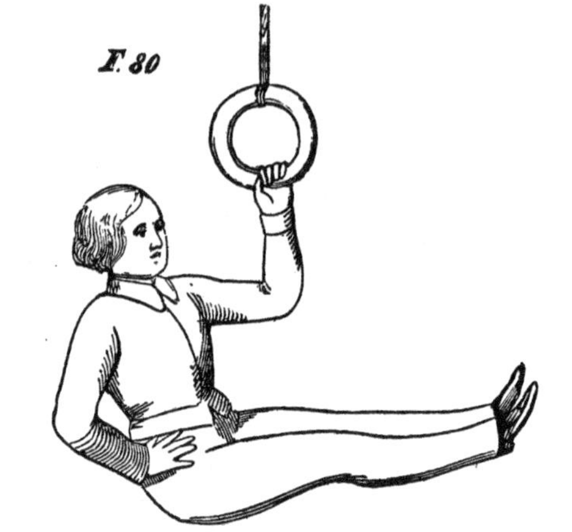

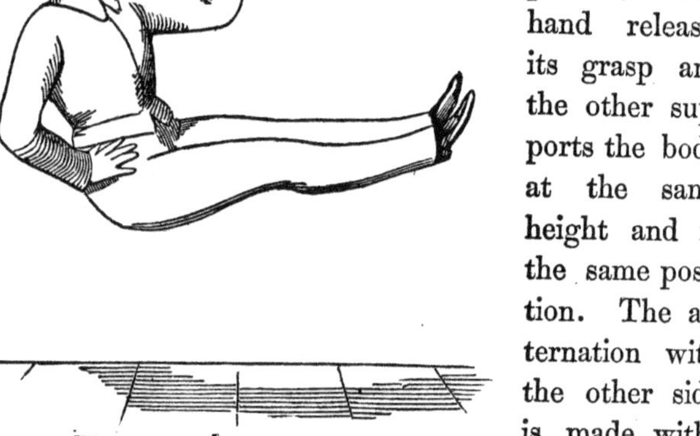

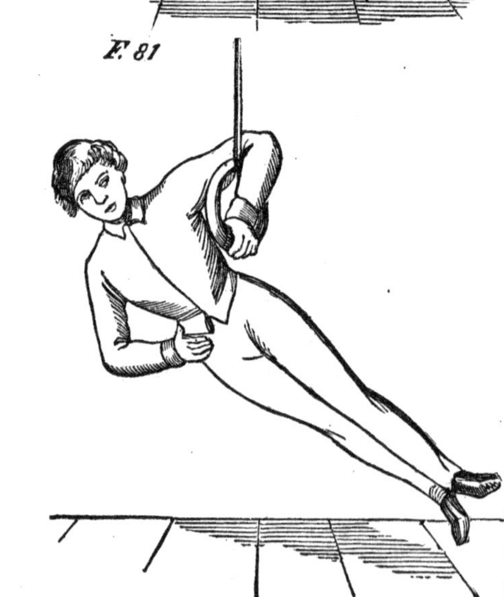

up to a horizontal line at a right angle with the body. As soon as this has been accomplished, one hand releases its grasp and the other supports the body at the same height and in the same position. The alternation with the other side is made without changing the attitude of the body.

Fig. 81. ANGULAR SUPPORT HANG WITH ONE ARM, *one, two, or three times.*

The rings at shoulder height are seized from the outside with the support grasp, in such a manner that the rope comes before the arm; for otherwise the arm could lean upon it and the exercise would be too simple and slight for this series. The body goes over into the support hang in such a manner that the transferring of the point of weight requires a powerful sidewise effort of the whole body.

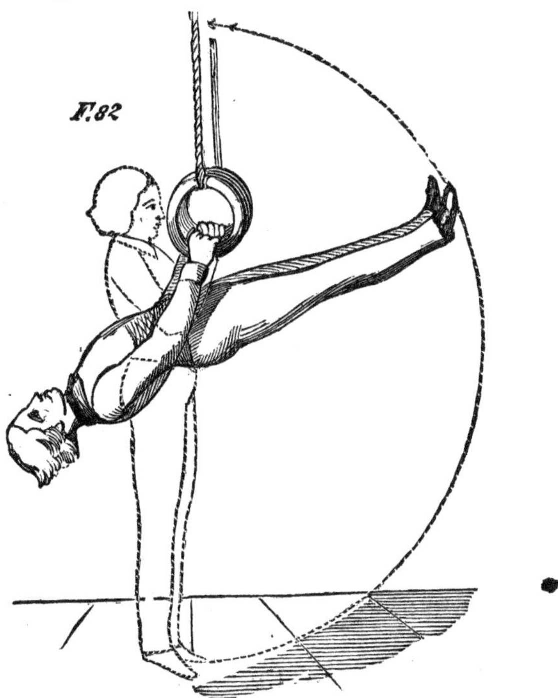

Fig. 82. RIGID DRAWING UP, *one, two, or three times.*

Rings a little above the head, are seized from the outside with the hang grasp. The pupil raises himself off the floor, then by an after movement a half summerset is executed, with the body kept rigidly straight. At no point is this rigidly straight attitude relaxed.

This is the essential point, and one can readily perceive the difference between the exercise as thus executed, and when done with a bending at the hip joint, be this bending never so slight.

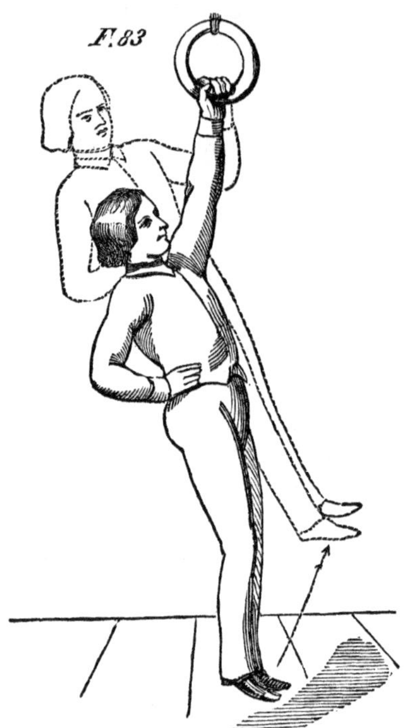

Fig. 83. Drawing Up Hang with One Arm, without Touching the Floor, *one, two, or three times.*

Seize the rings at the highest grasp point, and go over into the hand hang, with one arm stretched at full length. Now draw up the body until the arm is at a right angle. Both upward and downward the movement should be slow.

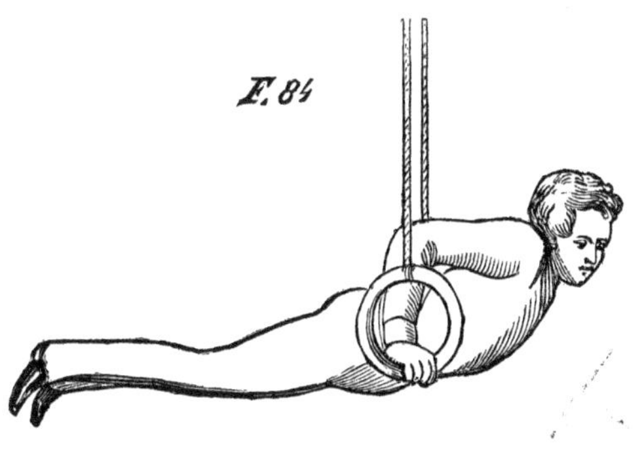

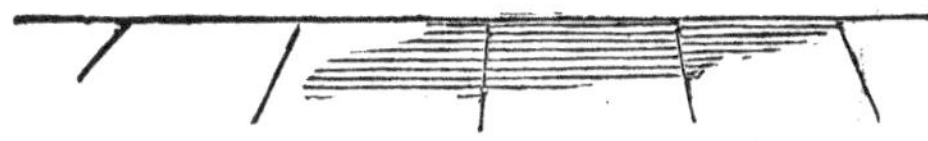

Fig. 84. SUPPORT WEIGHING, *during one, two, or three inhalations.*

Rings at shoulder height, are seized from the inside with the support grasp, and one goes into the support hang, (*Fig.* 14.) Thence by a gradual lowering and bending forward of the *rigidly straight body*, one goes into the horizontal suspended position, where it is retained. Through the action of the arm muscles the rings must be kept close to the body.

Fig. 85. HANGING BALANCE UPWARDS, *during one, two, or three inhalations.*

Rings as high as the head. Seize from the outside with the hang grasp, and go into the inverted position, (*Fig.* 54,) then keeping the body very straight, gradually and slowly turn it to the horizontal position and retain it there.

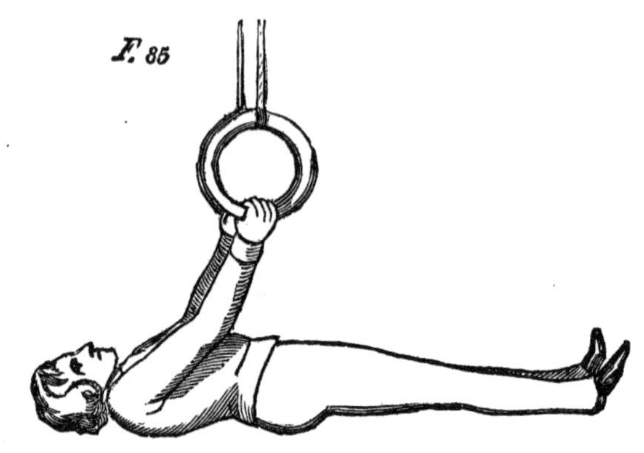
F. 85

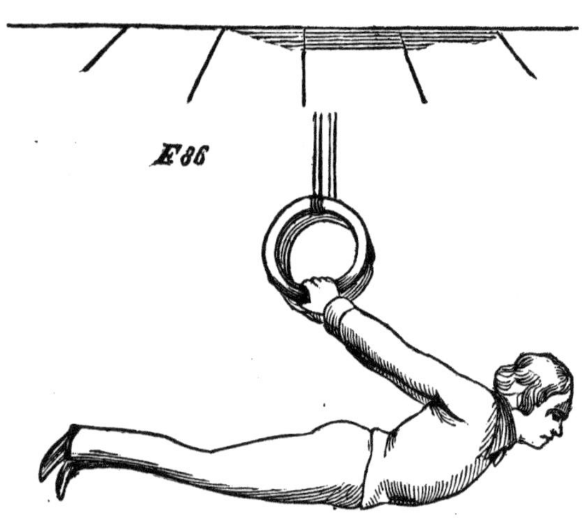
F. 86

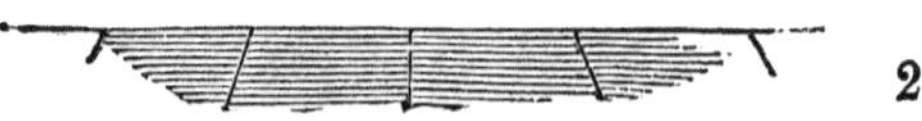

Fig. 86. HANGING BALANCE DOWNWARDS, *during one, two, or three inhalations.*

The same as the last exercise, except that this one has face down to the floor, the back being kept very rigid, and reaching the horizontal position, the body should be held there during the prescribed time.

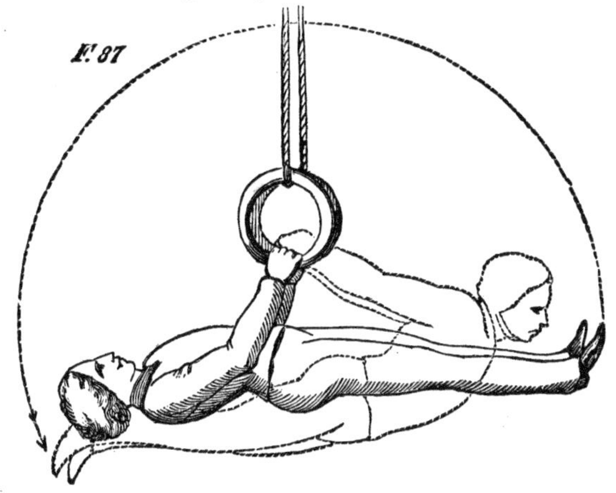

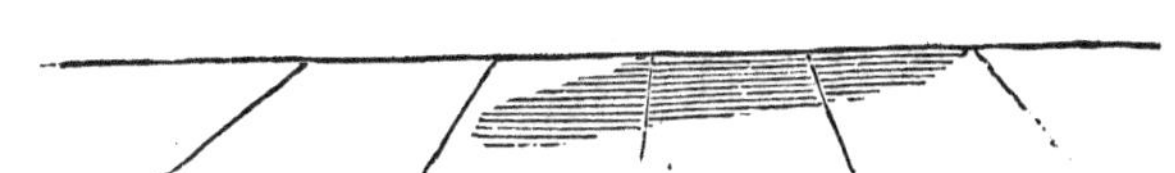

Fig. 87. DOUBLE BALANCE HANG, *one, two, or three times.*

The two previous exercises are united in this one. That of *Fig*. 85 is executed, then the transition is made to *Fig*. 86. The body should remain fixed upon reaching the perpendicular position, for a moment, for rest. This transition demands a high degree of power in the muscles of the chest, abdomen and back.

LEAPING EXERCISES.

The human body requires a variety of leaping exercises to complete a thorough gymnastic education. For the execution of these exercises no other apparatus is required than a simple cord horizontally suspended, and so arranged at the points where it is supported, that it can easily be raised and lowered, to determine

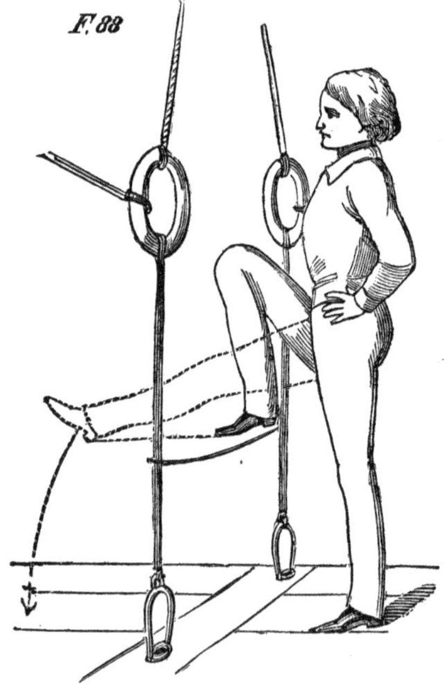

the capacity of the leapers. The straps of the Pan-gymnastikon are admirably adapted for this purpose, and are in fact superior to the ordinary wooden frame which is generally employed. The leaping cord can be attached to the straps with little metal weights slipped through the holes in the straps, or with small wooden pegs.

The leapers must come down on the toes with legs so bent that the head and spine will receive no concussion. If the leaping is done upon a floor, it is well to place a straw matting where the gymnasts are to land.

Fig. 88. FORWARD STEPPING OVER.

One places himself directly in front of the cord, and lifts one leg so high and in such a manner, that the leg from the knee down is in a perpendicular direction to the line of the cord, and can be stretched out over it without bending the body backward. Thus one places it on the other side of the cord upon the floor, and the other leg follows. In the same way the other leg now goes over first, so that each leg has the same exercise.

Fig. 89. SIDEWISE STEPPING OVER.

In a sidewise position, one stands close beside the cord, and raises the leg which is nearest the cord, exactly in a backward direction, high enough to be above the line of the cord, and over he steps upon the ground. The upper part of the body must resist the tendency to bend forward. The other leg now follows.

The higher one can place the cord the better. If one can keep the head and shoulders well drawn back, it is an improvement. The inclination to stoop forward, is of course very strong. As has been intimated, this must be resisted. This exercise exerts a happy influence upon the small of the back, and the hips. Persons affected with rheumatism or neuralgia in either of these parts, will find in this exercise a benefit.

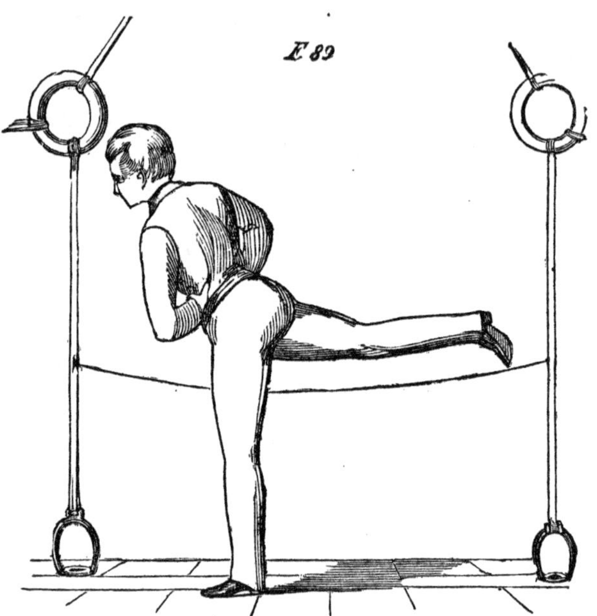

It should be added, though it is hardly necessary to mention it, that in the beginning the cord may be placed not more than eighteen inches from the floor. After many repetitions the cord may be raised as high as the entire length of the leg.

Fig. 90. Forward Leap.

Face the cord, and holding the heels together, leap over, keeping the two limbs in exactly the same position. The distance one is to stand from the cord, will be determined by the height of the cord—the greater the height, the greater must be the distance. The leap must be made from the toes. The knees must be well drawn up toward the chest, in making the leap.

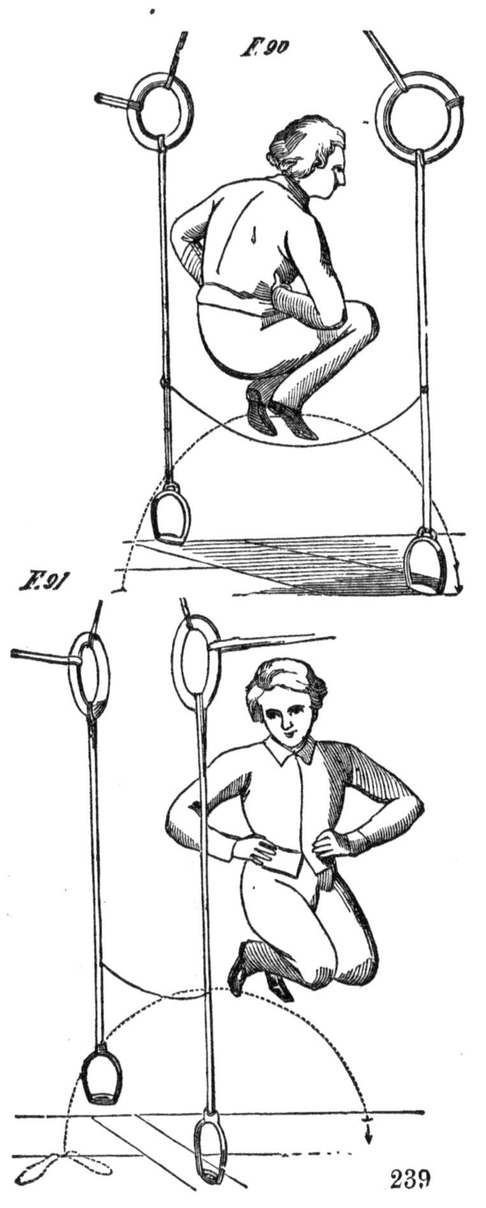
F. 90
F. 91

If this part be well done, the body need not rise much to leap a cord three feet high. And the body need not rise three feet to clear a cord five feet high. Persons with hernia, must exercise much caution in the performance of this feat. They ought not to do their best. In coming down on the opposite side of the cord, one should strike on the toes. If such a leap be well executed, so little noise is made that other persons in the same apartment will hardly hear the leaper.

Fig. 91. Sidewise Leap.

With one side close to the cord, and with the feet locked, leap over sidewise. Leap back in the same manner. The same rules in regard to the leap as in the last. This is a vigorous exercise for the muscles of the sides. Combined with the last, it will accomplish much for the longitudinal muscles of the back and side.

It ought not to be forgotten that these leaping exercises are very severe, and are pretty sure to be followed by soreness unless one is quite hardened to the work. Beginners should not make great leaps, but as it is supposed that those who practice these, have already performed all that precedes them, perhaps the caution is unnecessary.

Fig. 92. Twisting Leap.

As with the forward leap, the position is in front of the cord, with locked feet. One leaps forward and over the cord, in such a manner that with the leap the body makes a semi-circular turn or twist, and comes down on the other side of the cord, facing in an opposite direction. The same is now executed in an opposite direction; if from right to left first, it will be from left

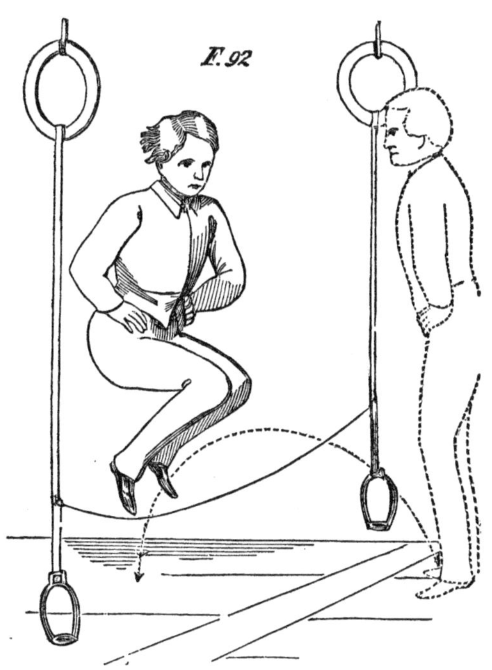

to right next. All exercises in which twisting the entire person, or the head alone, is a feature, are useful to those who are affected with vertigo. Not a few persons have been cured of dizziness by simply whirling on the heel.

Fig. 93. Sidewise Rigid Leap.

One stands sidewise toward the cord, and near to it. Leap from the ground so that one leg quickly follows the other, over the cord. During the leap each leg must be kept rigidly straight. Be sure to come down on the points of the toes. This exercise must be executed from alternate sides.

This will call for a vigorous exercise of all the mus-

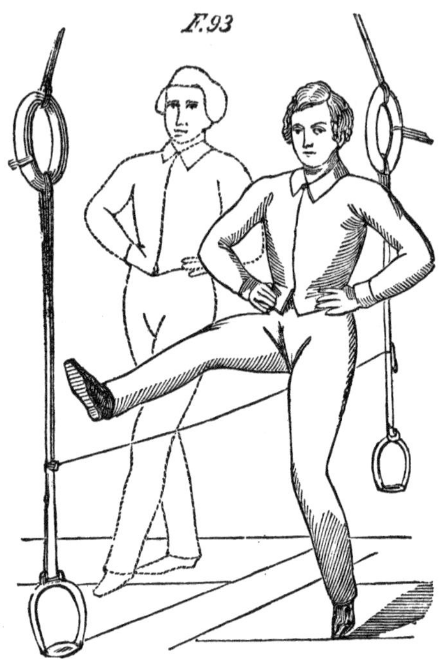

cles about the loins, abdomen and hips. At first it may lame the small of the back a little, but with care this will soon pass away.

Fig. 94. SPREAD APART LEAPING OVER.

The position and spring are the same as in *Fig*. 90, except the spring is quickly followed by spreading out the legs so they are apart at full width at the moment of passing over the cord, and are together again, when the points of the feet touch the ground on the other side of the cord.

In performing this feat, it is well to begin with the cord quite low. And every performer will be surprised to find how small the height he is able to reach in this

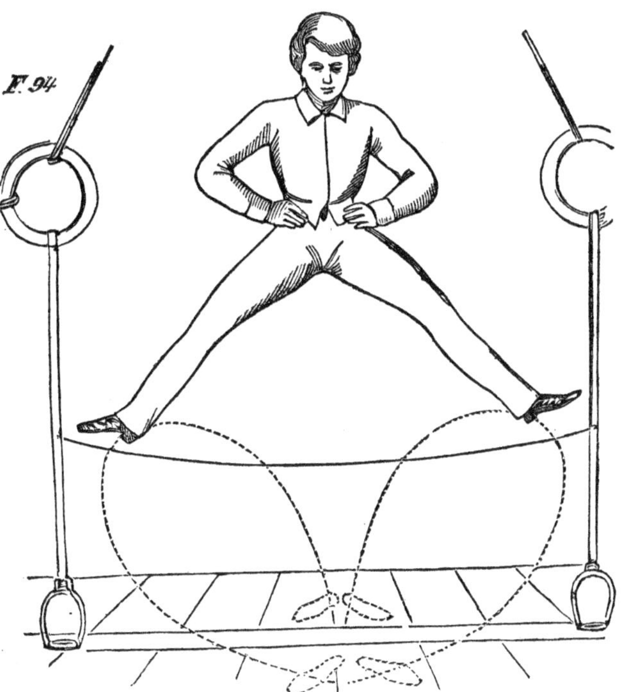

way. The high leaps are in great part achieved with the bending of the legs.

Fig. 95. BARRIER LEAP.

The rings are fastened at the sides as high as the hips. One of the hands seizes one of the rings from the inside. The spring with which one leaps over the cord, is made with the foot farthest from the grasping hand, while one braces himself upon the ring and keeps the body straight as it swings over the cord. Alternate from the other side.

One has a thousand occasions to use this leap. In crossing the fields, one has frequent necessity for leap-

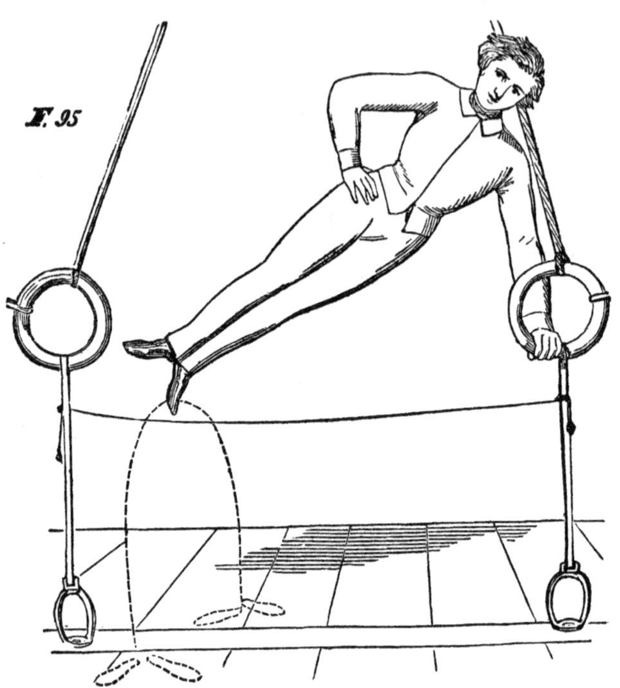

ing a fence, and as passing it in this way can be achieved even by an old man, if he understands the trick, it is recommended to all to practice this much. Leaping a fence in this simple and easy manner, not only looks well and saves time, but may save one's garments.

Fig. 96. Circular Leap.

This exercise consists of a leap, and at the same moment a circular twist, coming down at the place of starting. You must in landing reach precisely the same position that you had before the leap. The cut does not give a very perfect idea of this leap. It rather

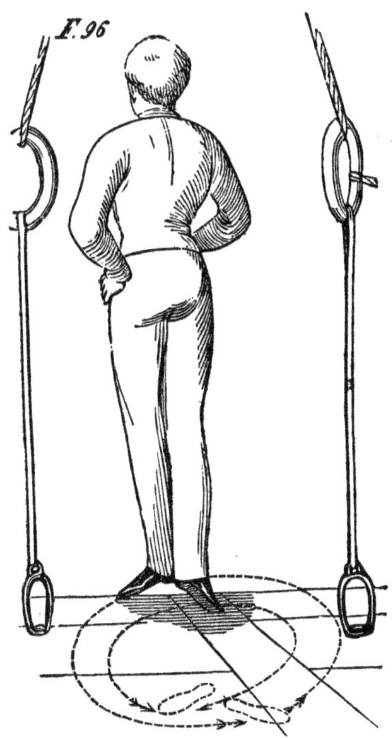

gives the impression that the performer has failed to reach the starting position. When the leap is made to the right, the left foot is placed twelve inches before the right, in position, before the leap is taken, and vice versa. This exercise takes place without the cord, and the only service of the rings and stirrups is to indicate the starting point. It is executed from alternate sides.

Fig. 97. SEIZING LEAP.

This exercise is for the purpose of learning how to seize firmly upon an object in the midst of a leap. At the moment when the body is over the cord in the leap, each hand seizes one of the rings, and holds tightly

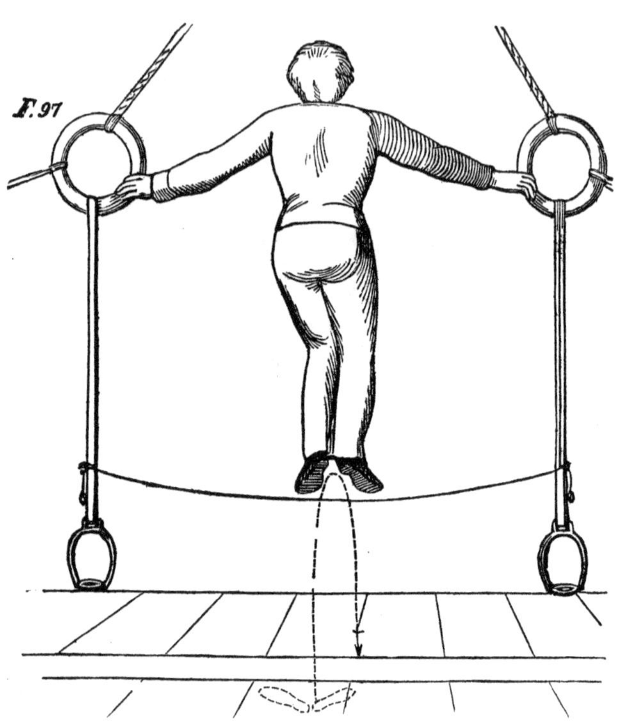

until he reaches the ground. This is executed without any tossing or swinging which might change the attitude.

This has the advantage of calling for quick eyes and hands. Indeed all these leaping exercises demand coolness and presence of mind. Those exercises which call for the use of muscles in a simple and unintelligent way, have comparatively little value. In a true development of the physical man, there must be an interweaving of the mind with the body, which can only be achieved by the practice of those exercises in which considerable skill is demanded. If the feats to be performed, do not require an active effort of the mind, the *man* is not improved. Holding one's self in the rings suspended as long as possible calls for a vigorous exercise of certain muscles, as does the lifting of heavy weights, but as there is neither skill or interest in either case, so there is little profit.

Many variations of the exercise represented in *Fig.* 97, will occur to every one.

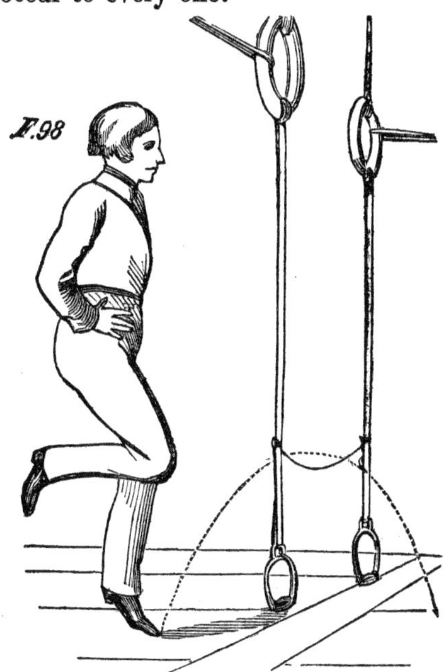

Fig. 98. FORWARD LEAP WITH ONE LEG.

Position the same as with other forward leaps. The body as close as possible to the cord. One leg is bent at the knee at a right angle, while the other executes the leap. Alternate.

Those who have been troubled with lame knees,

must practice this exercise with care. As there is a very severe exercise of the knee joint and the parts immediately sorrounding it, and as a lameness in those parts is apt to be a serious affair, too much caution cannot be exercised.

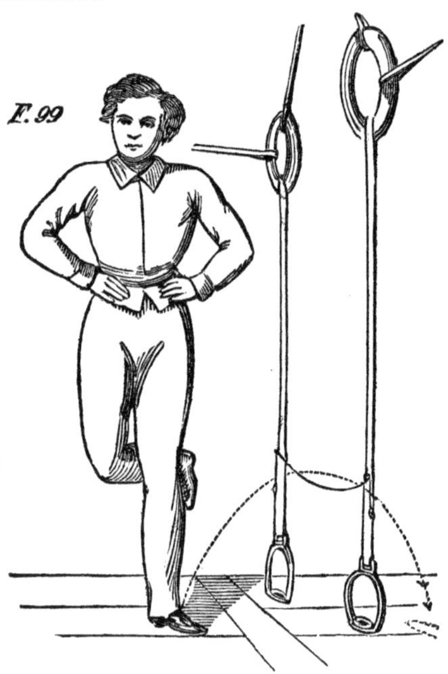

Fig. 99. Sidewise Leap with One Leg.

Like the last, except that one goes over in a sidewise direction, from a sidewise position, the leg that makes the leap being the one nearest the cord. Alternate the sides.

It might be necessary to repeat the caution given in the last, but as persons who have reached this point in these exercises have learned much by experience, and have likewise become tough, it is perhaps only necessary to express a general caution against undue exertions.

If there be deficiency in the left leg—if in size and strength it be inferior to the right, it is well in all the single leg exercises to give it more than half of the work.

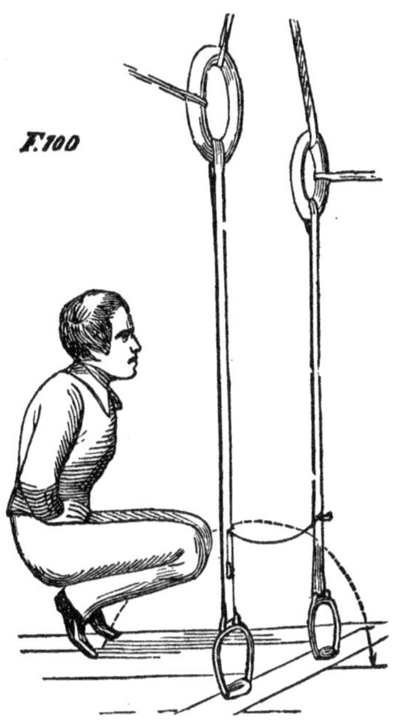

Fig. 100. SQUATTING LEAP.

From the lowest squatting position, with only the points of the feet upon the floor, one executes the leap forward over the cord.

This is an excellent exercise for persons with indigestion, torpid liver, or constipation. It will accomplish more in a single minute to arouse a vigorous action in the abdominal viscera than horse back exercise in half an hour.

Persons with hernia or hemorrhoidal tumors will, without warning, exercise due caution in the performance of this feat.

But in regard to this and other expressed cautions, if persons who undertake the execution of these severe leaping exercises, have performed in due course all the exercises of the Pangymnastikon which precede them, there will be little difficulty or danger in the execution of the most difficult leaps.

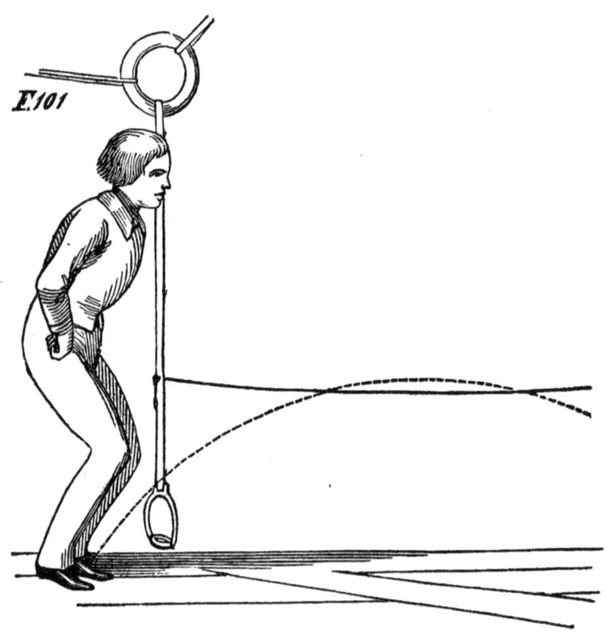

Fig. 101. OBLIQUE WIDE LEAP.

One takes his position near one of the straps and leaps in an oblique direction over the cord, coming down beside the other strap. This is to be executed from both sides, and alternately.

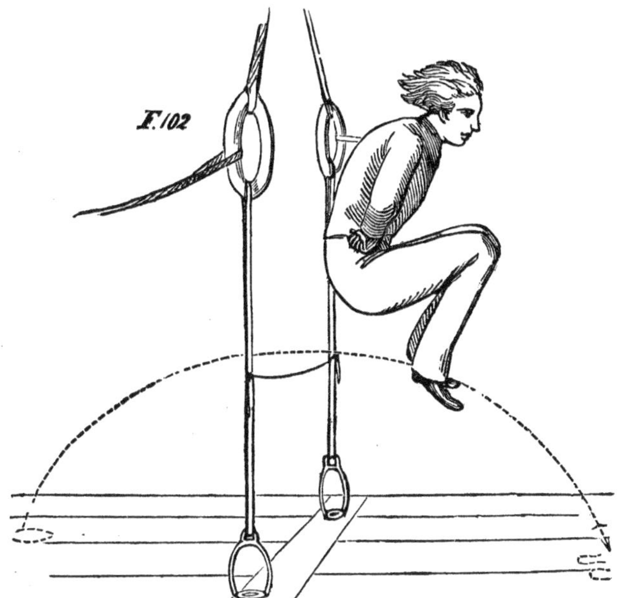

Fig. 102. Running Leap.

With a few short, quick steps, one must leap as shown in the cut. In the running leap it is the almost universal custom to spring always from the same foot. This must be avoided. Each foot must have its turn. One must always come down with the heels together, which is a general rule for securing safety and success in all kinds of high or wide leaps.

Fig. 103. Rising with One Leg.

In order to have the stirrup straps close to the hands as a reserve, in case the strength of the leg alone

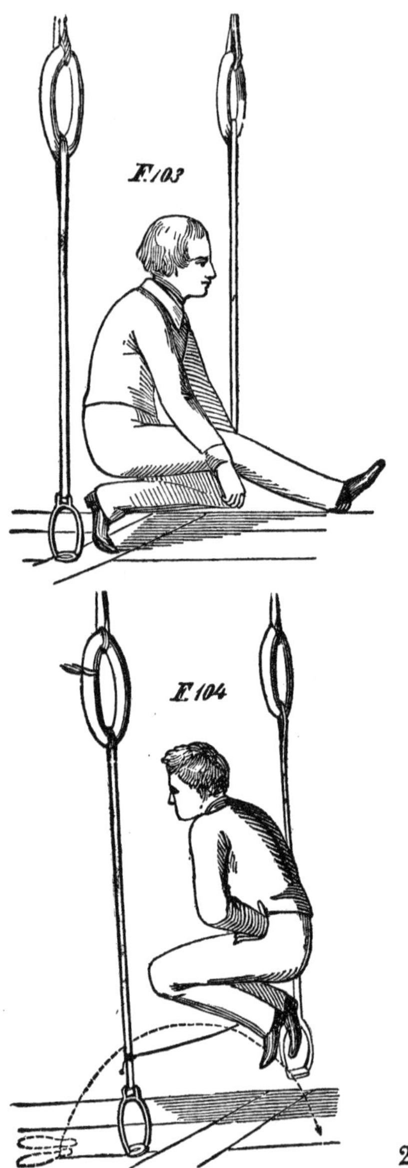
F. 103
F. 104

should not be sufficient, the rings are not fastened at the side.

Take a position between the rings in the lowest squatting attitude, resting upon the point of one foot, while the other leg is kept free and stretched out in front. Now rise to the erect posture, whereupon the other leg must take its turn.

Fig. 104. LEAPING BACKWARDS.

Stand with back to the cord, and leap directly backward over the cord.

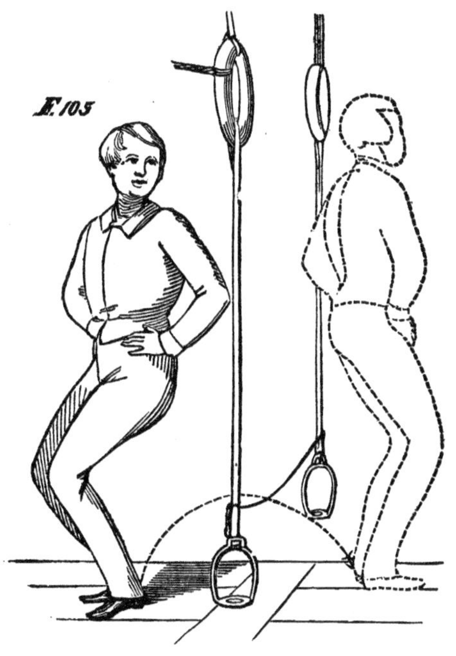

Fig. 105. BACK TWISTING LEAP.

Position the same as in the last. During the leap

turn half round and come down facing in the opposite direction. Alternate with turning the other way.

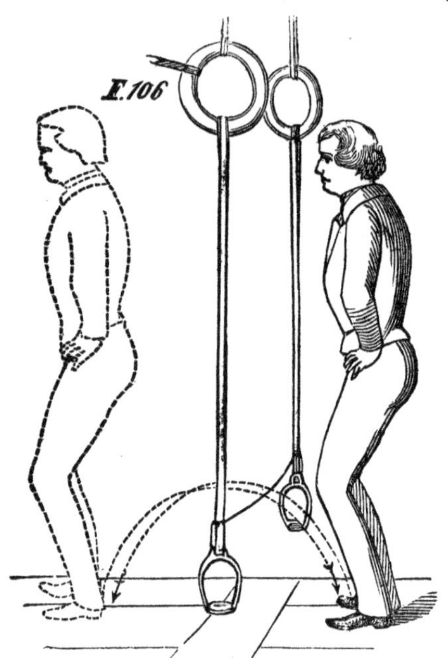

Fig. 106. OPPOSITE DOUBLE LEAP.

Execute the forward leap, (*Fig* 90,) and immediately follow it by the backward leap, (*Fig*. 104.)

This leaping forward and backward over the ropes, is, on the whole, perhaps the hardest of the leaping exercises. There can be no doubt of it, if you have had sufficient practice to enable you to leap about as high backward as you can forward. The faithful gymnast will be astonished at his improvement in the backward leaping. Beginning with the cord one foot high, he soon rises to two feet; then to three; and perhaps to four feet by the end of the first year. A much higher point than this even, may be reached by those, who, beginning with a fortunate composition, give a few moments every day to efforts in this department. Persons with hernia, unless well protected with a superior truss, must exercise great caution in the backward leap.

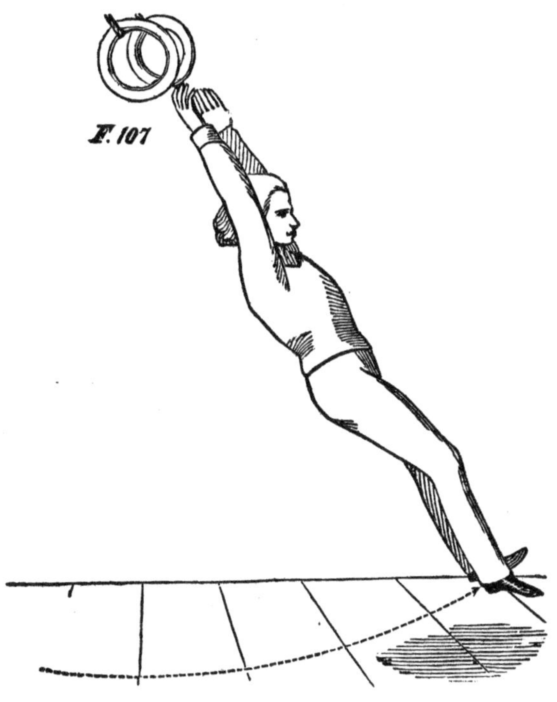

Fig. 107. LEAPING OFF DURING THE SWING.

At the end point of an energetic forward hand swing, let go of the rings, and come down as far forward as possible.

SUGGESTIONS IN REFERENCE TO THE USE OF THE PANGYMNASTIKON BY FEMALES.

This apparatus will be much used by females of all ages. Of the 107 exercises, there is not one which they may not execute with propriety and profit. I do not mean in a public gymnasium, but in the privacy of their homes. In order to secure the full enjoyment and benefit of the gymnastic exercises, they must provide themselves with the Zouave costume, such as is worn by the young ladies of the Zouave Military Clubs. The accompanying cut is a tolerably good representation of such a dress. It is cheap, easily fitted, allows the most perfect liberty to every limb and muscle, while it can be put on or thrown off in a single minute.

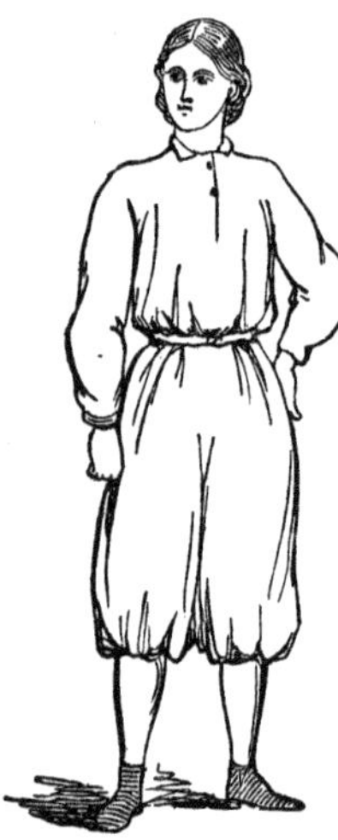

When a lady is done with her morning cares, and would dress for dinner, she slips on her Zouave, and stepping to the Pangymnastikon, devotes a few minutes to its exercises. It may be put up in almost any bed-room, and thus she may enjoy the strictest privacy. In putting it up in a parlor, study or bed-room, the walls need not be marred, while it can be taken down and removed out of sight in a single moment, nothing remaining but several comely hooks.

FIRST PRESCRIPTION.—FOR GIRLS AND WOMEN.

When you would dress for dinner (though it should

not be within an hour of that meal) on Monday, Wednesday and Friday, execute one to ten inclusive, each exactly the given number of times. When the hour indicated is not convenient, just before retiring at night is the next best hour. Do them precisely in the order prescribed, and on the days indicated. Do not look up other exercises and attempt them. Follow the prescription as faithfully as you would that which advises doses of medicine. Practice this prescription during one month. A marked improvement in the manner of execution will be developed during the month.

SECOND PRESCRIPTION.—On Monday, Wednesday and Friday, when you would dress for dinner, execute eleven to twenty, exactly the number of times indicated in each exercise. Try hard every time to perform each exercise better than before. Continue this prescription during one month.

THIRD PRESCRIPTION.—On the same days and at the same hour, execute twenty-one to thirty, during one month.

FIFTH PRESCRIPTION.—On the same days and at the same hour, execute twenty to thirty, during one month.

SIXTH PRESCRIPTION.—Same days, same hour, one to thirty, during one month.

SEVENTH PRESCRIPTION.—Same days, same hour, thirty-one to forty-five, during one month.

EIGHTH PRESCRIPTION.—Forty-six to fifty-nine, one month.

NINTH PRESCRIPTION.—Thirty-one to fifty-nine, one month.

TENTH PRESCRIPTION.—Sixty to seventy-five, one month.

ELEVENTH PRESCRIPTION.—Seventy-six to eighty-seven, one month.

TWELFTH PRESCRIPTION.—Sixty to eighty-seven, one month.

After one year, select from any of the series such exercises as are most agreeable, and perform them at pleasure.

It will be observed that nothing has been said of the exercises from eighty-eight to one hundred and seven. These are leaping exercises.

The leaping exercises may be used, ad libitum, after entering upon the third prescription. It is only advised, that whenever the back is made to suffer, greater caution should be exercised.

FOR CHILDREN OF EITHER SEX, THE PANGYMNASTIKON IS ADMIRABLE.

Children of either sex, as early as four or five years of age, may begin a course of Pangymnastic training. The course I have advised for women, I would prescribe for children. The leaping exercises they will practice with great pleasure and profit.

FOR MEN OVER FIFTY YEARS OF AGE,

I would prescribe the same order of exercises. Permit me to assure you, gentlemen, that much of the rigidity of muscle, and inflexibility of spine and limbs, which you think inseparable from your age, may be removed by a course of mild and varied gymnastic training. I hear you say that "gymnastics are for young people, not for old folks like us." I believe no class of persons would be more benefitted by proper physical training, than that class of American gentlemen who, having led active business lives, have, in advanced life, retired to sit down and enjoy themselves. The characteristic stoop of the shoulders, among the aged, could be prevented by a few very simple exercises frequently practiced.

For Large Boys, Young Men and Middle Aged Men,

I would advise the following course:

First Prescription.—*Every morning* before breakfast, about an hour before dinner, or some time during the evening, execute one to fifteen. Continue this one month.

Second Prescription.—Sixteen to thirty, one month.

Third Prescription.—One to thirty, one month.

Fourth Prescription.—Thirty-one to forty-five, one month.

Fifth Prescription.—Forty-six to fifty-nine, one month.

Sixth Prescription.—Thirty to fifty-nine, one month.

Seventh Prescription.—Sixty to seventy-three, one month.

Eighth Prescription.—Seventy-four to eighty-seven, one month.

Ninth Prescription.—Sixty to eighty-seven, one month.

Tenth Prescription.—One to forty-five, one month.

Eleventh Prescription.—Forty-six to eighty-seven, one month.

Twelfth Prescription.—One to eighty-seven, one month.

Use the leaping exercises at pleasure from the beginning.

Follow the above prescribed course during one year, and then continue the exercises in the Second and Third Series, ad libitum.

When any man has followed the prescribed course for one year, and then continues the use of the Pangymnastikon a few minutes every day, it would be safe to insure his health at very low rates.

The clergyman with sore throat, who shall follow this course, will need neither nitrate of silver nor a journey to Europe, to cure his bronchitis.

The victim of Dyspepsia, Chronic Headache, or Rheumatism, will find this road leads directly out of the valley of sorrows.

Persons of either sex, and of all ages, will find in the faithful practice of the Pangymnastic exercises much of health and strength, and such an increase of days as will more than a hundred fold compensate for the time devoted to this truly great invention of the distinguished Schreber.

SCHOOL DESKS AND SEATS.

A radical change in school furniture is imperatively demanded. The seats and desks, now in vogue, compel an attitude which must result in a stooping form. The other day I stood an hour on the street, and saw more than five hundred persons pass. Not one was erect. Bending over the desks in our schools, ten years, would make us crooked if we were composed of spring steel.

The desk top must be so arranged that it may be raised nearly to the perpendicular before the face of the pupil, and the book held in a position which shall compel him to sit with head and shoulders well drawn back.

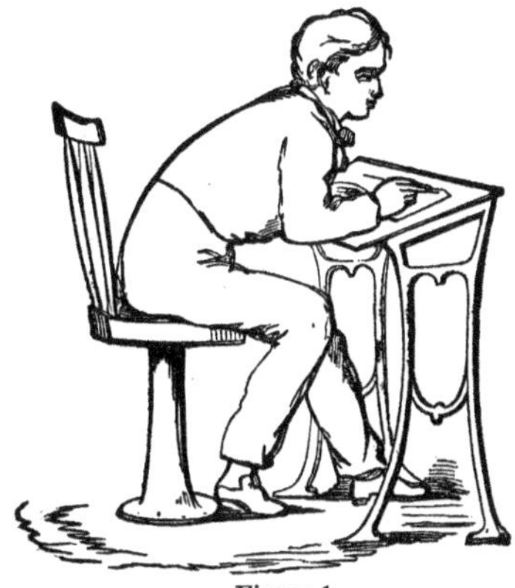

Figure 1.

Fig. 1 exhibits a fruitful source of our characteristic stooping shoulders.

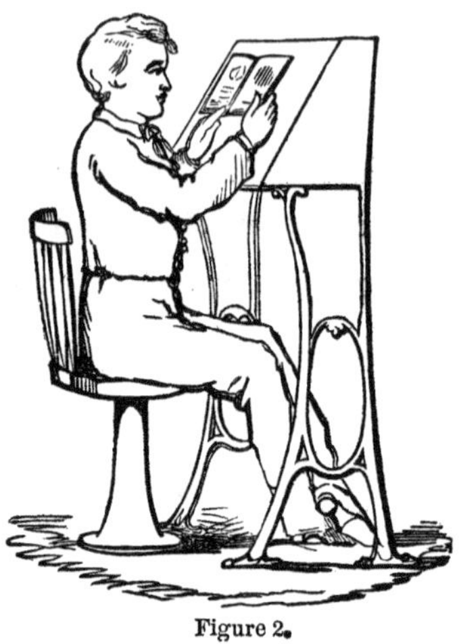

Figure 2.

Fig. 2 presents a better desk, and the change of position in the pupil.

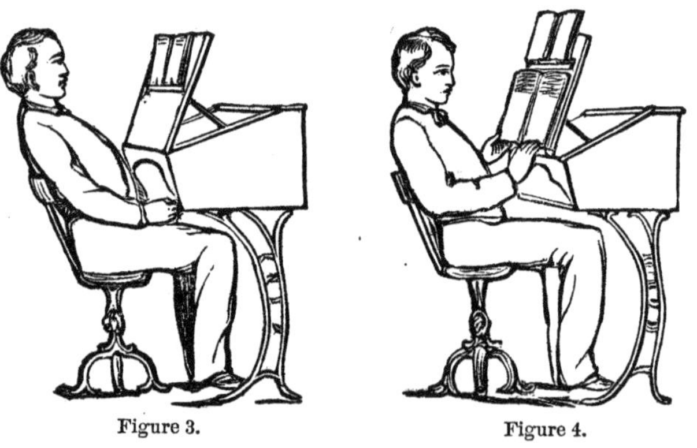

Figure 3. Figure 4.

Fig. 3 is a model desk, meeting every want. The top can be raised to any height that may be desired, or let down nearly horizontal, for writing exercises. On the desk top, it will be observed, is a bar which supports the book. This can be moved at pleasure, and has a pair of fingers which will hold the book in any position.

Fig. 4 shows *two* support bars, an arrangement which must prove most grateful to students of the languages, and to all others who have occasion to consult a dictionary while reading. The seat is likewise adjustable. It can be raised or lowered several inches by a single motion of the hand.

The ordinary desk may, at a trifling cost, be changed into the new one.

THE NEW BOOK HOLDER.

A book holder has been invented which will be used in schools upon the desk already in vogue, and in private houses upon the common table.

The "Holder" is seventeen inches high, and eight inches wide. The cut gives a good idea of it. A very simple arrangement enables the pupil to raise and lower the book, which is held in any position by a pair of fingers. The support bars are armed with small hooks, with which they are hung upon the cross rounds. A "reader" may be held on the upper bar and a dictionary on the lower one. By a simple means the holder can be brought up more or less immediately in front of the face, so as to compel the student to sit very erect or allow him to bend forward more or less.

This book holder cannot get out of repair, is very neat and cheap, and if made of rose-wood and silvered

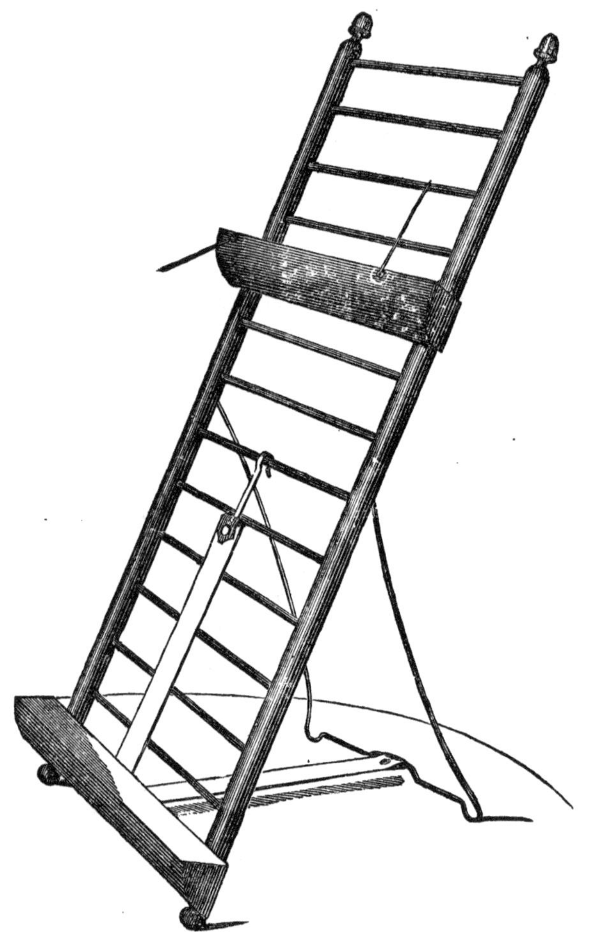

wire, is exceedingly beautiful. A patent has been applied for.

VENTILATION.

An unventilated gymnasium is an absurdity. We visit such an institution for health, and not for mere show of muscle. At least such is the fact with people of brains, A gymnasium without apparatus would be regarded as a failure; a gymnasium without ventilation is a nuisance.

Sanitary science involves no problem so grave, and heretofore so difficult of solution, as the ventilation of our houses. We live most of the year within doors. A pure atmosphere is indispensable to health. We must live in an artificial heat. How shall this heat be supplied, and the air of our houses constantly changed?

An open fire is without doubt the only effective means heretofore employed. Although not economical, it is, for many reasons, most satisfactory. It fills the house with sociability and a sense of comfort, and secures a complete ventilation. But the great waste of heat, with the dirt and dust, are objections which are greatly lessening the number of open fires. Besides it would not be easy to warm a large hall or church with this means.

Furnaces are rapidly multiplying. Nearly all private dwellings of any considerable size are supplied with them. A great variety have been invented.

Their essential differences lie in their various capacities for the production of heat from a given amount of fuel. All, so far as I have been able to ascertain, have essentially the same facilities for ventilation; the heat in each case being introduced at the floor, and escaping at or near the ceiling. Without doubt the needed change of air can be secured in this way, but it is not less certain that the great mass will refuse to bear the waste. The heat, upon entering the room, rushes immediately to the ceiling, and if there be an opening there, escapes, without having been felt by the persons who may be sitting in the room. In an apartment heated by a furnace, the difference between the upper and lower stratum of air is something wonderful. At the floor our feet are cold, and the children are cautioned against lying down lest they take a cold, when, if you climb to the ceiling, the heat may be suffocating. To make openings in the ceiling and allow this heat to escape, while persons are sitting below in the cold, is certainly a wasteful policy. If all the dwellings, in any American city, were furnished with the facilities for ceiling ventilation, I do not believe that five in a hundred would be ventilated during the damp and cold seasons of the year. The great mass would not consent that the heat, which they have paid for at the coal yard, should leave without touching them. So the windows and doors are made as close as possible, and the people live without ventilation. The consequences are most lamentable. Before the invention of stoves and furnaces, headache, catarrh, bronchitis and consumption, were comparatively rare.

Many years ago, in discussing the subject of ventilation, I said, "If, while sending a thousand cubic feet of heated air into a room, we could take the same quantity of cold air from the lower part of the room, we should have a perfect ventilation." But at that time I had no idea such a feat were possible, unless it were accomplished by air pumps, which should force the cold air out and thus bring the heated air down. But nothing in the mechanical world is impossible with the Yankee. The result, which I thought impossible, has been achieved by some live Yankee, and by a means so simple, that, as usual, it is wonderful that some one has not thought of it before. I have examined the invention and seen it well tested. I will try to explain it. The furnace is a good one I believe, and is placed in the cellar like others. The heat is conveyed to the apartments above in the usual way, and in brief, the furnace is, so far as I know, in the departments of generating and distributing heat, not unlike other furnaces. Some advantages are claimed for it by the inventor, but as I do not know him, and have had very little opportunity to examine other furnaces, I have in this department no opinion to offer. In regard to the ventilating department, however, I entertain a very decided opinion. In a hygienic point of view, I am confident it is one of the most important discoveries with which I am acquainted.

To illustrate it, I will suppose we have a single apartment to warm. A furnace is placed under it. A pipe conveys the heat in at one corner of the room. At the opposite corner is a register, which, in appearance, is not unlike that through which the heat enters the room. This is known as the ventilating register. From it a pipe runs back to the furnace, and enters the chimney with the smoke pipe. The result is, that the heat passing up the chimney creates a strong draught in the ventilating pipe, which of course must be supplied from the lower stratum of air in the apartment above. The cold air taken out at the floor, compels the heated air from the upper part of the room to descend to the floor. A remarkable comfort and economy are thus secured. When a piece of paper is burned, or a cigar smoked near the ventilating register, the smoke descends and quickly passes through the register instead of rising into the upper part of the room.

The purity of air in the room, and the warmth of the feet, attracted my attention before I knew that the house, in which I was visiting, was warmed by a furnace of peculiar construction.

This is a truly beneficient discovery. I confidently believe it will contribute much to the health of the American people.

When the autumn returns, I shall introduce one into my gymnasium in Boston. This furnace is known, I believe, as the Eagle Right-Angle Ventilating Furnace. If any body can invent a better one, and will satisfy me of its superiority, in a future edition of this work, I shall be happy to announce it.

The subject of ventilation is one of such paramount importance, that both in the Gymnastic Monthly and in future editions of this book, I shall introduce all that promises to give the people a purer air.

THE NORMAL INSTITUTE FOR PHYSICAL EDUCATION.

This Institution was incorporated in 1861, and is located in Boston. Its Board of Directors includes many of the most distinguished of our New England educators. President FELTON was its active and earnest presiding officer, up to the time of his death. The departments of *Anatomy*, *Physiology* and *Hygiene* have able professors; that of *Vocal Culture* is in charge of Prof. T. F. LEONARD. Dr. DIO LEWIS has charge of Gymnastics.

This Institution is the pioneer in a new profession. Men and women of enterprise and industry, will find in this field *health*, *usefulness* and *large profit*. The full course continues ten weeks. During the year there are two courses—the first beginning on the 2d of January, the second on the 5th of July. A circular can be obtained by addressing Dr. Dio Lewis, Box 12, Boston.

At the two "Commencements" of the Normal Institute, which have already occurred, eminent educators were present and made brief addresses. The following extracts are made, as indicating the interest among this class of persons :—

"Dr. Lewis has solved the problem. He has marked out the way. Many eminent teachers are pursuing it with the most excellent results. We recognize the debt due Dr. Lewis. He has done us teachers and our pupils a vast amount of good."—*D. B. Hagar, Pres. of the Am. Institute of Instruction.*

"I am now satisfied that Dr. Lewis has found the true scientific process for physical development. It was my privilege to welcome Dr. Lewis at his very first arrival here, and everything since then has only confirmed my confidence in his ability to superintend the work."—*Rev. Dr. Kirk.*

"Henceforth we shall delight to think of Dr. Lewis as one who holds our welfare very near his own; we shall turn to him for sympathy and encouragement in our failures, and shall love to bring our successes to him, as belonging more to him than ourselves."—*Valedictory of the first Graduating Class, by Miss May.*

"I rejoice, Mr. President, that the Normal Institute for Physical Education has been established in Boston. I rejoice that it has at its head a gentleman so admirably qualified to give it eminent success. I believe that no individual has ever, in this country, given the subject of Physical Education such an impulse as has Dr. Lewis. He deserves the credit of it.

You may not know it, ladies and gentlemen, but this Institution is famous in every part of the land. There is not a live educator in America who is not looking to see what is to be the result of Dr. Lewis's Institution in Boston. These exercises can be introduced into any school-room with desks. The problem is solved.

I trust, ladies and gentlemen, that this is the commencement of a new era, and that the system taught by Dr. Lewis, will be universally introduced into our schools.—J. D. PHILBRICK, ESQ., *Superintendent of the Public Schools of Boston.*

Managers of educational establishments will find among the graduates of this Institution teachers of a system of gymnastics, marvelously full of interest and variety, admirably calculated to impart symmetry, grace, flexibility and strength, while some of the graduates have had long and varied experience as teachers in schools for intellectual culture. Several who have held honored places in Seminaries of learning, seek, in adding physical culture to their labors as teachers, to restore lost health.

I may add that a great many exercises which are much used in our gymnastic classes, do not appear in this volume. I would not discourage efforts to introduce gymnastics with the assistance of the book alone, by those who cannot avail themselves of the advantages of the Normal Institute, but it is doubtful if any body ever learned to dance well with only a book for a teacher; and when we add two hundred difficult exercises with the arms to our elaborate exercises of the legs and feet, and at least one hundred skilful combinations of the two, we do not go too far when we advise all who would teach successfully to avail themselves, if possible, of the advantages of the Institute.

This work, it is hoped, may introduce physical culture to a thousand schools, which otherwise might enjoy no advantages in this department of education. The field is large, and as yet in a great part unsurveyed. To this I shall add other volumes. As already announced, I shall publish several considerable volumes devoted to the Movement Cure, and as soon as it seems to be needed, I shall add a volume upon School Exercises.

THE BLOW GUN AND SPIROMETER.

A system of physical training, adapted to the wants of the American people, must involve much special, direct training of the respiratory apparatus. Our national weakness is found in the chest. A tabular statement of the deaths by consumption in America, is frightful. The coughs heard every where, are distressing. The subject has deeply interested me.

The Blow Gun is a good means of enlarging and strengthening the chest, and its use moreover so amusing that it does not require a conviction of duty to impel one to its use. It is so simple, that with a word of explanation, it may be made by any worker in metals. The barrel is thirty inches long and half an inch in the bore. It is of copper, and made perfectly straight and smooth within. Outside it is lacquered. The mouth-piece is an inch wide, fitted to the lips, and silver-plated. The arrow is of wood with brass ferule, and metal point which passes with a screw through the entire length of the wood. A tuft of camel's or goat's hair is attached to the back end. A target with the bull's eye, and four rings, completes the preparations. The target is shown.

The company divided into squads of four, sit on either side. One squad steps into position, and each person slips an arrow in at the mouth-piece of his gun. Holding the gun with the hands placed, as upon the ordinary musket in the act of shooting, the captain cries "make ready," and each one fills his lungs to their utmost capacity, then "take aim, fire!" The arrow is blown with great force into the target. The squad, in order, marches away, the captain announces the result of the shot, and a squad from the other party takes its place on the "mark."

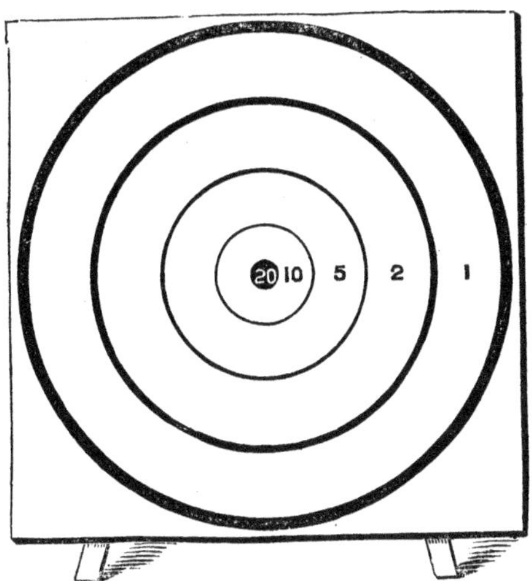

All the interest which attaches to the ordinary target shooting, is found in this blow-gun target shooting, and the lungs receive a very happy training. They are enlarged, and the respiratory muscles strengthened.

The SPIROMETER is still more effective. This instrument is very beautiful, resembling a highly finished small-sized clock, and will adorn the walls of any parlor. It has a pair of hands which are connected with the internal mechanism. A mouth piece at the end of the tube is applied to the lips, and the lungs being filled to their utmost capacity, the breath is forced into the instrument. With the utmost exertion but a very small amount of air leaves the lungs, for the reservoir receiving the air, will not hold more than an ounce. And it will be readily perceived that all the power with which the air is forced through the tube, is simultaneously felt in every part of the lungs. In the uttermost corner of the lungs the entire pressure is felt. If the instrument were capacious enough within to receive a large part of the air in the lungs, then instead of the air being forced into every cell, the cells would be closed as the air was forced out. But in the use of this instrument, when the lungs are completely inflated, the effort to force the air into the reservoir is simply an effort to force the air into every air passage and cell, for the pressure is as great backward as forward.

The lungs contain millions of air cells. In our artificial life, many practices—tight dress, bad position, etc., close many of them. Consumption begins with this closure. Keep them open and consumption cannot begin.

Filling the lungs to their utmost capacity, and applying the lips not *around*, but against the mouth-piece, you blow with a force sufficient to carry the hand to 100. Do this every day for a week. The second week you can blow hard enough to carry the hand to 150. And as the strength of your respiratory muscles increases you will be able to force the indicator up to 400.

I repeat that the lungs being always fully inflated, the effort to force the indicator around the dial will be sure to drive the air into every air cell. Nothing but disease *already established* can prevent the air from finding its way into every cell. With this accomplished, and frequently repeated, it is simply impossible for consumption to make its first deposit.

The Spirometer cannot get out of repair, and is an exhaustless source of interest to one's self and friends.

UNIFORM WITH THIS VOLUME.

WEAK LUNGS

AND HOW TO MAKE THEM STRONG:

OR,

DISEASES OF THE ORGANS OF THE CHEST,

WITH THEIR

TREATMENT BY THE MOVEMENT CURE.

Profusely Illustrated.

BY DIO LEWIS, M.D.,

AUTHOR OF "THE NEW GYMNASTICS FOR MEN, WOMEN, AND CHILDREN."

In One Volume. Price, $1.25.

TICKNOR AND FIELDS, Publishers.

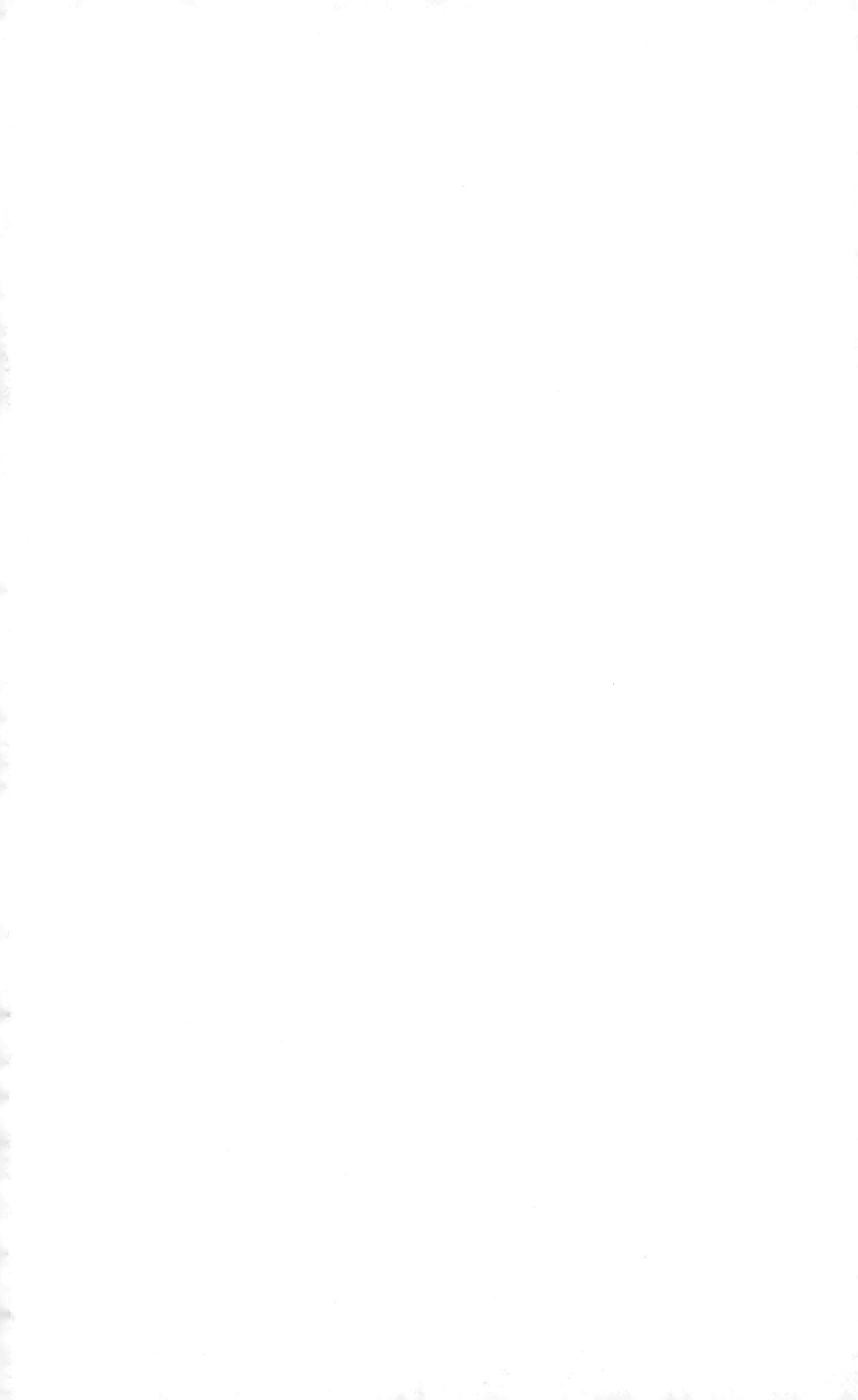

www.ingramcontent.com/pod-product-compliance
Lightning Source LLC
LaVergne TN
LVHW010232110826
845151LV00004B/1275

* 9 7 8 1 4 2 5 5 2 4 8 9 0 *